TRAINING
FOR
LIFE

A Prescription for Fitness

HERNANI OURIQUE

FriesenPress

One Printers Way
Altona, MB R0G 0B0
Canada

www.friesenpress.com

ISBN
978-1-03-911947-5 (Hardcover)
978-1-03-911946-8 (Paperback)
978-1-03-911948-2 (eBook)

1. *HEALTH & FITNESS, EXERCISE*

Distributed to the trade by The Ingram Book Company

Table of Contents

PREFACE

WE LIVE IN A world where access to information is so easy to come by. A couple of minutes scrolling on your phone enables you to learn so much about one subject that you feel like an expert. This gold mine information, however, puts us in a position where many of us create a bias around what is the right or wrong thing to do. Information doesn't equal knowledge, and the one particular area where I would love to intervene and add my expertise is fitness. I often try to display lots of empathy when I hear certain things like, "squats are bad for your knees" or "we should never be doing deadlifts."

I believe people who make comments such as these are often misled. What you are telling me with comments like the above is that sitting on your toilet is bad and picking up your kids is something you should never do.

Another thing that doesn't help are the people we should trust in the industry who make ridiculous claims. I get it. It sells. It brings attention. Attention pays well.

There is so much contradictory information out there and people are often suffering from paralysis by analysis—this frustrates me. It frustrates me because I sincerely care about YOU and YOUR health. I don't know you, but you deserve to know simple and actionable ways to better yourself without needing to go to extremes.

There are so many books out there on powerlifting, bodybuilding, running, and thousands alone on various diets. I don't recall coming by any that just focus on ways to maintain longevity. That is my goal with this book. I want to offer a different approach on how you can make lifestyle changes that realistically fit your day to day.

As of now, what you are about to read are my thoughts on how to approach fitness and health for longevity. Each year, we learn more and more about the human body and what is potentially optimal for our health—with new knowledge, more experience, and strong science my mind can change. This is important because you must challenge any current beliefs you currently have about fitness and health. What I often find is that the solutions are simple, not easy.

Master the elements in this book and you will be a true ambassador of training for life... and for that I would like to say, thank you for choosing fitness.

LOOKING FORWARD

WHEN YOU ARE EIGHTY years old, what will your goal be? Have you even ever thought about yourself at that age? I'll tell you my goal: I want to be able to take out my own trash. Why? For starters, you probably need to or it will overflow. Let's think about the process there is to taking out the trash. You pull the bag out of the bin—sometimes it needs a nudge to pull it out—then you tie it up and carry it out front, walk down a few stairs open the garbage bin, and toss all the garbage bags inside, all while waving hello to your future neighbour and talking about how nice the weather is. I would love to do all of this without worrying about falling down the stairs or getting winded from potentially going back and forth for a few trips. To me, performing this simple task an elderly age has always been a level of independence that I aspire to when I'm older.

This goal is one I share with as many people as possible and the reaction is usually the same. They seem to appreciate how simple and distant it is. What is funny to me is no one questions whether the goal is achievable. If I said I want to become a professional athlete, I'd typically get a look of doubt. Why? Is it really that easy to take out the trash at 80 years old?

Why look forward?

From a young age, I got used to helping out my grandmother who had suffered from a subdural hematoma when she was in her late 40s. A subdural hematoma is when blood starts to collect between the skull and the brain. This can cause severe headaches, which is one of the symptoms my grandmother was feeling. I still remember the day I got home from school and saw two paramedics in my grandmother's room, with my mom by their side. My grandmother was such a hardworking woman. She was always up, out and about, and very energetic until this incident happened. She ended up in a coma state for about ten days.

Her life changed forever. The subdural hematoma took away her ability to be independent and move around on her own unless she had her walker. I would go to the store for her, moved items that were relatively heavy for her, and sometimes we would walk and she would hold on to me for balance to go from point A to point B. That's when I started thinking about longevity at a young age. Ask any of my family members: I was quite an annoying kid, usually shaming people for smoking or doing things that weren't necessarily good for them. Some of them insisted that I will do the same one day... still waiting.

When you grow up helping someone else at a young age, you can't help but think about how unfortunate it is that a simple task such as going to the washroom is now a chore that is not only physically but also mentally fatiguing. This made me start looking around more when I was out and about and seeing things through a different lens. I started noticing the amount of work people in their 60s had to delegate because they simply couldn't complete the task without risk of injury or were simply limited by their physical capacity. At the same time, shovelling snow and mowing lawns for that crowd is precisely the reason I made a few bucks as a kid. So maybe it was a win-win at the time.

Let's consider the opposite. I am sure we all know someone late into their age who looks like they have more energy than you do; they are up early and doing more in a day than you can imagine. They have the ability to hike up steep mountains in the morning, do some yard work in the afternoon, and mess around with their grandkids before they enjoy some quiet reading time. These same people usually brag about how much fitter they are than their own kids—you would think with age they would become humbler.

What separates these groups of aging folks from each other? What makes one thrive into their old age while the others just survive? What about that uncle you have heard about who lived to one hundred despite chewing cigarettes? How did he make it there? The answer is not that sexy. Instead, there are a number of factors as to why someone can live a long, happy, and high-quality life. There are ways to "build a hedge" (think of this for now as your emergency fund; we will dig into this in a later chapter) against just surviving in life and truly enjoy your time on earth into old age. I am excited to show you how in the following chapters.

My grandmothers baseline fitness went from being able to run, jump and carry relatively heavy objects to being stuck in a bed for months and having to relearn everything. It has been eighteen years since that unfortunate event and if you saw her today you would see she stands most of the day, cooks and cleans, walks around taking small steps and uses a walker or someone's help for longer walks. She is fitter today than she was eighteen years ago when she was in her coma. Those with lots of life experience who hike in the morning, do yard work, and then play with their grandkids have "built a hedge" against just surviving so that they can continue to be independent. They remain to be fit today. What do they have in common— they continue to focus on a lifestyle that promotes movement, they aren't doing it to be Olympic athletes, what is it that they do? They train for life.

READER EXERCISE 1—Get Your Walk On

Throughout this book, I have included readers' exercises related to the chapter. Some might be actual physical tasks or mental tasks, which will hopefully start to create some good habits towards your lifestyle.

Walking is something a lot of us take for granted. I have seen multiple people around me lose the ability to walk on their own. They either need assistance for balance from others or from objects like ski poles or a walker. When I train or think of people like my grandmother, it reminds me how thankful I am that I can simply get up and walk to wherever it is I want to go.

The first task is quite simple. Go outside and walk briskly for twenty to thirty minutes. I would like you to hold a conversational pace for the duration of the walk and enjoy your surroundings.

Post a picture of you on Instagram after your walk: use the hashtag #trainingforlife.

LONGEVITY

L ONGEVITY IS DEFINED AS the length of your life. The average life span of a human varies based on where you are located in the world, genetics, access to food, clean water, health care as well as some other variables. According to the World Health Organization (WHO), the average global life expectancy from the year 2000 to 2016 increased by 5.5 years. Since the average has gone up, some parts of the world are still seeing chronic diseases affecting more people, which leads us to believe that medicine, clean water, and access to food has been paramount in helping us push our life expectancy up. The question then becomes, how many people sixty to eighty years old are independent and living a high-quality life?

That's what I mainly want to focus on—anyone who has access to clean water, food, and healthcare already has more than most humans who once walked/still walk this world, and we should be grateful for that. However, nobody wants to become sick. Though some unfortunate circumstances do arise, there are still actions we can take to minimize risks of becoming ill or one hundred per cent dependant on others to live and survive.

With that being said, we seem to be doing great at living longer, but how can we do it better!? How do we thrive as we age to enjoy what is around us!?

Perspective

In the summer of 2018, my partner Sam and I went with a friend to Algonquin Park Provincial Park in Ontario, Canada, to hike, explore, and of course take pictures for Instagram (it is very beautiful and I highly recommend visiting). In one day, we covered just over thirty kilometres hiking up and down trails, some steep, some rocky, some muddier than others, but each one equally rewarding. It was amazing to see so many people of different ages during each hike. Everyone always walked by with a smile and didn't hesitate to say hello. There were the occasional noises, which spooked my friend and me since we grew up in the city. Apparently, we find alleyways more comforting than forests.

After this short trip, I remember talking to Sam about how grateful I felt that we could cover so much distance in a day, just on a whim. The idea that we didn't have to worry about our ability to walk up and down rocky hills or about our energy levels to cover that much distance in a day.

Fast forward to 2019, and I am sitting around a table with my family on Terceira, a small Island in Portugal where I was born. Next to us was a lovely couple we had met who were touring the Island, trying new food, exploring the underground caves, and everything else the island has to offer. After our short conversation with them, Sam overheard the couple talking about how we looked fit and that if they wanted to continue living their lifestyle, they would have to consider introducing more fitness into their routine.

I loved hearing that because they said something I try to preach often: they wanted to use fitness as a tool to support the lifestyle they enjoy. They looked down the line at a distant horizon and recognized that if they want to continue doing what they love, they were going to need to budget time to focus on their health. I hope they are still enjoying their travels today.

Keys to lifelong health

What are the training secrets to longevity? Honestly, you have might of heard of some of them, and I will touch base on topics such as sleep, stress, strength, and others. Studies that seem to contribute to a high-quality life usually seem to fall into five main categories:

1. Cognitive health—healthy brain

2. Core strength—strength through the midsection
3. Grip strength—hand strength
4. Leg strength—force of your thighs
5. Fast-twitch muscle fibre development—power and speed

1. COGNITIVE HEALTH

When it comes to exercise, we always think about the body, but the mental benefits are quite incredible and, in my opinion, often overlooked in the general fitness space. In college, we had a class named Special Populations, which covered topics such as training those with cardiovascular disease, pregnant women, respiratory diseases, etc. The top of the list for what can help people in these categories was always exercise. Whether it was for helping with anxiety, decreasing damage to the brain, or personal fulfillment, exercise has massive benefits for mental health. There are correlations to those who stay fit and active throughout their life and how their mind functions in relation to memory, mood, and just the ability to "be sharper" up top.

That being said, to keep the brain healthy, exercise is one way: food, relationships, stress and so many other factors are important to keep in mind and we will address some of them throughout the book. Sam (my better half) and I are always testing each other in some capacity to remember things, and play card games at night to force us to challenge our brains in a way that is fun.

Challenge: Grab a friend and learn a new card game; then master it.

2. CORE STRENGTH

Core strength is very important for longevity. Many people tend to focus on the core for vanity purposes, which usually leads to only focusing on the abdominals only (front side). But your core is 360 degrees, which includes not only the abdominals but also your obliques (sides) and erectors (back). You use it every day from the first sit up you do out of bed to the groceries you have to carry. When the core is strong, the body as a unit becomes stronger. How do you know if your core is weak? If you find your back aches after standing or sitting for a long time, it can be an indication that your core is weak.

These muscles are vital in helping us maintain independence throughout our lifetime. Whether you want to be physically dominant or physically competent the importance of core work has held true in the world of fitness and health for many years. If you want to do a fun test (be safe!) go stand in front of a wall, and give the wall a little push with your hands while keeping your feet locked down—what muscles did you feel? An issue that is common among older folks is falling due to lack of balance, coordination, reflexes and, yes, a weaker midsection. We always want to work on "natures belt."

Challenge: Get into the top of a push-up position (tall plank) with your arms fully extended on the ground and holding yourself on your toes. How long can you hold this for while keeping your body straight? If you can hold it for more than two minutes, try it again after two to three days, but this time on your elbows.

3. GRIP STRENGTH

Many overlook grip strength: the ability to which you use your hands and essentially hold on to various objects. Think of it as the strength in your hands and your forearms' flexors (inside) and extensors (outside). This type of strength can come in various forms such as open palm, closed palm, pinching, and fingertip (think rock climbers). Some researchers have found that this is a reliable way to determine your true biological age, which is pretty cool! Just like core, grip strength is required in everyday activity. Think about picking up your kids, carrying groceries from the car to your home, or when you are holding on in the bus when the driver thinks he is rally racing.

Challenge: Here is a fun grip test. Find a sturdy tree branch or a bar, squeeze it tightly with your hands, then slowly pick your feet up off the ground and see how long you can hang on. Time yourself. In two to three months, try again. If you can hold on longer, chances are that your grip got stronger.

4. LEG STRENGTH

When I say leg strength, I am not just talking about the muscles that lay on the front and back of your legs such as your quadriceps and hamstrings, but also your glutes, which support the hips. This is such an important area to focus on. Not only for strength, but mobility as well. Strong legs are important to having independence as they literally let us stand up and get out of bed. I like to look at very simple examples of leg strength when it comes to longevity, which is your ability to stand up from a chair, or even more difficult, the ground. A person who has stronger legs has a much easier time standing up from a fall, as it requires you to put emphasis on the front of the leg to get up. Something a lot of us take for granted is having the ability to stand up from various positions.

Challenge: Set a timer for sixty seconds and see how many times you can sit and stand from your chair. Or count how many times you can go from lying on the floor and getting back up *without* using your hands. How many repetitions can you do?

5. FAST-TWITCH MUSCLES

Muscles are extremely important to us. They allow us to perform everyday movements such as sitting, standing, walking, dancing, playing the guitar, and anything else you can think of. We have two types of muscle fibres: slow twitch, also known as Type I, and fast twitch, known as Type II. Think of slow-twitch muscles (Type I) as your everyday walking muscle; you aren't moving fast but you *are* moving. These muscles have incredible endurance and can contract for many repetitions. You can look at a marathon runner and be pretty confident she has well-developed slow twitch muscle.

Fast twitch (Type II) is your ability to sprint, react fast. The "I am helping someone lift a very heavy couch" type of muscle. These muscles are great at creating forceful contractions of the muscle and give us the ability to do things quickly, which is exactly why fast-twitch muscles are so important to think about when aging. Why? Well, as we age this is the type of muscle that starts to decrease in size if it isn't attended to. Because these muscles help us with sudden bursts of energy, they can play a huge role in preventing accidents that require us to react quickly. I had a teacher who told me the first thing he teaches someone who enters a nursing home is how to stand up from a fall. We can prevent those worries of falling by staying strong.

Challenge: Want to test how explosive you are? Okay! First, be safe—find a place where you won't get hurt and try a standing long jump. Position your feet directly underneath your hips, do a partial squat, and jump forward and land in a partial squat for three attempts. How far did you go?

I believe if we look at these five points and start to expose ourselves to them, we will have a pretty solid foundation of what it takes to become more resilient with the life we have, whether that is physically or mentally. Some of us will look at it and say great, I am going to do some planks, squat, carry things, jump, sprint, and challenge my brain on a regular basis. Do that on a consistent basis, and I am happy. Others might go further down the rabbit hole and that is pretty cool too.

The payoff

On that same summer trip to Terceira Island in 2019, there was a moment that brought me lots of happiness as a son once worried my mother's health. There was a time where my mom was smoking regularly, wasn't moving much, and she wasn't always making the best choices to support a lifestyle that would benefit her long term. As her only son, this concerned me because if anything happened to her, it would now be up to me to take care of her, which I would do in a heartbeat. But this made me realize a truth that her actions are not only doing her a disservice, but potentially in the long run… she could be doing her family a disservice. This sounds harsh, but if I imagine myself as a father, I never want my kids to worry about me; I want them to know that I can take care of myself into my old age. I instead want them to say "Great… Dad took his shirt off again."

Before I move on, I want to give you my point of view on what my mother's health looked like years before one of our trips to Terceira. My mother told me she had been an athlete growing up, but we all know that doesn't really mean anything during adulthood. She was always a hard worker, but when it came to her physical health, I was always quite concerned. From my view, I would think things like, "Will she see me get married?" "Will she get to see her grandkids?" The reason I thought these things was mainly because of the way my mom treated her body.

Knowing what I know now, I am aware the body is pretty resilient, but I have seen lots go wrong as well. I didn't want that for my family, let alone my own mother. But slowly over time, as I egged my mom on to change, it was when she started taking care of family members who needed it, she changed. She ate better, let go of the cigarettes, and started to use her body more frequently.

Now... one of my uncles in Terceira is a sound engineer. As part of his job, he sets up the stage for anyone who performs in front of a crowd. There were warnings of a bad rainfall coming, so around 12:30 a.m. we got a phone call from him, asking for help to take down the stage and all the equipment to avoid water damage. My mother and I went to go help. To make things worst, this was all on a beach. There was so much equipment that needed to be moved, and most of it was not light at all.

My mother was energetic the night my uncle called. She was packing, lifting, and carrying this equipment from the stage to the parking lot. Some of these involved what looks like a farmer carry, which is simply holding something in one or both hands, or carrying something while hugging it, a lot of items had an awkward grip and some team work was needed. This was all done on sand, by the way, which makes this so much harder. If you have never carried something in the sand, pick up a heavy water jug and try walking across your bed. Not easy.

Each trip to the parking lot was roughly 150 to 200 feet on a slight incline. The men at first were saying to my mom, "Miss, please. This is too heavy for you" only to watch her have fewer issues, while taking no breaks, compared to the other people who were there to help. Afterwards they were saying, "Nobody mess with her; she is strong." And things like, "I should start going to the gym."

You see, my mom had a strong enough core to protect her spine. She had a solid grip to carry these awkward items, and her legs could pick up whatever was in her way. She did this quickly and definitely had mental gratification that she is strong and proved to others that just because she is a woman she is not weak and fragile. All of this happened for a couple of hours. I was proud of her.

That worry I had had about my mother's health and future independence growing up... it disappeared. That one night, I saw someone who was the best version of herself that I had ever seen. She is "younger" now than she was many years ago. She didn't win a championship trophy or set some crazy personal record—all she did was help out a family member at an odd time. Is there any better sign of strength? She did something I preach a lot about to anyone I work with. Apply your fitness somewhere other than the gym.

READER EXERCISE 2: Gimme Five

Take the five categories that contribute to longevity I mentioned in this chapter and do them all! When you complete the challenges, write down your results somewhere you can find them. Repeat them again after 60 days to see if you have improved.

1. GET MENTAL: Find a friend and play a game that challenges your mind! I recommend a memory game such as Concentration, a game you play with a standard deck of 52 cards, where you try to create matching pairs. You start by laying all the cards face down, and on your turn flip over two cards. If they match, you take them out. If they don't match, flip them back over but try to remember where they were in case you flip a similar number on your next turn.

2. CORE: Max effort plank! Get on the floor, propping your body on your toes and elbows while holding your back straight and still. See how long you can hold that position! It might be seconds or even minutes.

3. GRIP STRENGTH: Find a tree branch (make sure its sturdy!) or a bar and hang off of it for as long as you can! If you can't hold your bodyweight yet, simply lean back so you pivot from your heels while you hold on to that branch! When your grip gets tired, make sure to step back with one foot to avoid falling.

4. LEG STRENGTH: Put on a sixty-second timer and sit on a chair (or on the ground), then stand up without using your hands!

5. FAST-TWITCH MUSCLES: Standing long jump, start by placing your feet underneath your hips. From here you will go into a partial squat while swinging your arms back behind your hips. You will then swing those arms forward as you push through your legs and jump as far forward as you can while trying to land softly in a partial squat. Try this three time and record you furthest attempt.

Post these tests or games on your Instagram: use the hashtag #trainingforlife.

FITNESS OUTSIDE OF THE GYM

STARTED LIFTING WEIGHTS AND focusing on training to become a better athlete. At first, it was to become a better soccer player. Shortly after that, I redirected my focus to the sport of CrossFit®, also known as the "Sport of Fitness." When it came to results, what I typically looked for was: Can I jump higher? Am I faster? Am I beating the competitor beside me? Can I add more weight to the bar? I was asking myself these questions to make sure that I was improving. After a while, I wondered something: How effective am I outside of the gym? Coaching many people made me realize that most people, for the most part, don't actually care about their personal records or if they are beating someone else. They care about daily function and enjoying their life outside of the gym walls.

Use real life to measure your fitness

A client of mine relayed a story that really pushed my perspective on this topic. We were hanging out after a class and he was telling me about his measuring stick to indicate how he knew he was getting fitter. He had a brother living in the United States near some great ski hills. Instead of using the chair lift, they would hike up this hill, clip up at the top, and work their way back down. The first time they went up, he took about two hours to hike to the top with breaks due to fatigue. When they got to the top, he needed to rest roughly forty minutes just to feel ready to start making their descent. To make matters worse, he didn't really enjoy the trip down as he was tired from the hike up.

After training for some time at my gym, he mentioned how after a couple of years, he can now hike up in about 40 minutes (the time it took them to recover previously), rest for five minutes, and have a great time coming back down the hill. How cool is that? All because he was fitter. He got to enjoy an experience that he previously couldn't because of his personal work capacity. This doesn't change just who you are physically but your self-confidence goes up dramatically as well.

This got me thinking… he wasn't using weight on a barbell to determine if he got better; he used an outdoor activity and his subjective feelings to indicate if he felt like there was an improvement. The question I like to ask now is, How many people are missing out on something they enjoy or want to experience simply because of their well-being? I don't have a real answer, but from people I know in my personal life, I can count too many.

Now, I am aware not everyone really cares about hiking, snowboarding, or playing sports, but this applies to other aspects of life as well. Are you tired after playing with your kids? What does walking up a flight or two of stairs feel like? Could you run 400 to 600 metres to chase someone who stole your phone? Think of any scenario you could potentially be in during your lifetime… now, do you want to be limited by how you can react to it?

One Friday afternoon, I had a track session at a local park near my house, and I had a series of running intervals to complete. I remember finishing my session off with three sets of 800 metres around the track in a certain time. Now, during one of my rests, I saw two teens walking towards my bag acting strange, but I didn't really think anything more of it. As I started my final set of 800 metres, I got to about the 200-metre mark, so I was on the complete opposite side of where I had my bag. As I was turning, I looked and my stuff was gone!

I fired up the jets and bolted for the corner of the park, which has three large flights of stairs and that's where the teens saw me as they tried to flee while throwing my stuff everywhere. They crossed the street and a driver in a pick-up truck saw that I was chasing them down, so he stopped traffic to let me safely run across the street. Within about two to three seconds after crossing the street, the first teen knew he was not going to outrun me, so he gave up and handed me my bag, which I pulled out of his hand. The other teen came back and I made him lift his shirt and pull out his pockets to make sure he didn't have anything valuable to me.

After I gave the teens a life talk, I walked away, relieved that I had all my stuff and annoyed because they had interrupted my training session. But they might of also help me set some sort of record on whatever distance it was that it took me to catch them. I knew one thing that day: I was fast and speed had helped me, thanks to training.

Pro tip: Don't steal from people sprinting on a track.

Trust your feelings

The reason people don't really use their subjective feelings to determine their fitness during random events like the one I just described is for three reasons: it's not always measurable, it's not always repeatable, and it's not something you can take a video or picture of and post on social media. These are very real-life scenarios that happen every day. They need to be talked about more, though, because that is what we do most of the time. We carry things and often reach down and pick things up, so we need to be a functioning human if we plan on being an independent human for a long time.

Using life as a metric is much more effective for ninety-nine per cent of people, especially in the developed world. Not everyone wants to deadlift 501 kilograms like Thor Bjornson, who is an Icelandic strongman, also known as the character "The Mountain: in *Game of Thrones*. Nor does everyone want to run a sub two-hour marathon like Eliud Kipchoge, a long-distance Kenyan runner who broke the two-hour mark for 26.2 miles in 2019. I mean it: some of us sincerely don't care about those feats of performance, although they are very impressive. Some of you might like the *idea* of deadlifting that much or running that fast until a coach presents what it takes. Others with the right genetics, geography, and work ethic will get very close, but again, way more people couldn't care less.

Some people just want to walk pain-free and have more energy throughout the day. There is absolutely nothing wrong with that. Now, a bit of discipline and guidance is still needed to achieve those goals, but if we are open about our "why" then a lot of pressure can be taken off versus looking at the best of the best in the gym or sporting world, which can be intimidating for those who really do need a dose of exercise in their life.

I once saw a coach post up a workout program. In the description, it mentioned how this is not for the ninety-nine per cent: Only the tough shall survive and only those willing to make sacrifices were worth his time. For the most part, that's fine because I believe each coach can choose who her target audience is, but something about it didn't sit right with me. These programs often put out are great if you can learn a thing or two from them. But I am usually concerned for those who see them and think that's what it takes to achieve great levels of fitness. These programs are really effective at peaking your fitness by having you train at what is usually an unsustainable approach. As fitness writer Coach Dan John says, "After a peak is a cliff," which means down you go. What we want to do is give you a program that allows you steady progress over the long haul and not for just twelve weeks. Have you ever done a thirty-day challenge and then fallen off completely? That's the cliff.

These programs are usually actually *completed* by… you guessed it: the one per cent. What a great program—one where only a handful of people benefited from it. I find that sets the majority of people who truly want to see a difference in their health at a loss and put in a position that makes one think the only way to being fit or getting healthy is to do what the one per cent are doing. Nothing is further from the truth; you do not need to do what elite athletes do to see benefits. You need to do what works best for you, in your life, in your current situation which changes all the time. Even though many people hate it, change is the only thing that is constant and therefore we must adapt.

1% to 99%
I follow a set of athletes and coaches on Instagram who were once competing at a high level in CrossFit®. They were in the top one per cent; this required them to train multiple hours a day and complete many different tasks for the sake of being better at exercising faster. It so happened to be that these athletes started having newborn babies around the same time, and like most people who have babies, their lives changed. Things became busier and their personal Instagram feed started preaching a different

message about balance, but in a motivational and inspiring way to keep fitness alive. (Not surprisingly, they are now part of the ninety-nine per cent, figuratively speaking).

Once the worldwide COVID-19 lockdown occurred during 2020, they started posting about them coming together over Zoom calls and doing what they called "Dad Sessions" at 5 a.m. before the kids woke up. Sometimes it was comedic to see one of them post that they had to cut their session short because a baby woke up. To me, this was very inspirational because that time is not ideal for top-performing athletes to train, but because that is no longer the goal from my understanding, it was the best they could do to fit their new lifestyle. Their priorities are now running businesses, raising a family, and I am sure other things, though I do not know the full context of their lives.

Just do something!

The reason I like enjoy following these athletes as an example is because they "get it"—they know that something is better than nothing, they know doing three sets of squats and doing three rounds of their planned five-round workout (because baby is crying) is still going to push the needle forward. They went from sacrificing time and energy to train for a sport to now training to supplement the kind of life they want to live.

We can make any plan we wish for in this wonderful thing called life, but you never know when your physical capabilities might stop you from doing that, whether that is your ability to hike up the ski hill with a sibling and enjoy every bit of it, whether you are trying to keep up with your kids, or when you need to catch those thieves stealing your stuff while you are doing some sprint intervals at your local track (shakes head). These things are hard to measure. But they are things that happen every day and I'm sure you want to enjoy the world and the experiences that it has to offer everyone.

What happens in the gym is temporary and these often are not the memories you remember, but that time you carried your Dad into the hospital because he injured his leg is something you will never forget. Yes, this also happened. Lots of people laughed as I carried a grown human like a baby. My dad works on high-rise buildings and he was essentially trying to swing his leg over a beam. As he was rotating, he tore one of the ligaments in his knee. He called me up and said, "Hey, I need you to pick me up; I just hurt my knee." Without hesitation, I put whatever I was doing aside and drove down to his job site. There he was, limping away as one of his coworkers tried to help him.

I had a small Honda Civic at the time, and he is a pretty tall dude so putting him in the front seat was not going to happen. Instead, we got him into the back seat so he could keep his leg outstretched. When we got to the hospital entrance, I helped him out of the car. Then I tried helping him to walk but his limping didn't make it any easier. The first thing that came to my mind was, "You do loaded carries all the time; just pick him up." So pick him up is what I did. I don't know how this affected him emotionally, having his son carry him like a teddy bear, but it was much easier on my part, and it makes for a funny story. Now, what I did in the gym that day, I don't remember.

READER EXERCISE 3: 30/30 Run

Whether you are someone who is just starting your fitness journey or someone who loves to live in the four walls of a gym, I challenge you to take your next workout outside. Grab some friends and go to a park or a trail. Spend five minutes warming up with a light jog and some leg swings going forwards and backwards, side to side. Once you are all warmed up and ready to go, I want you to jog/run for thirty seconds and then walk for thirty seconds for a total of fifteen rounds (fifteen minutes). For an extra challenge, run uphill!

Post a picture of you and/or your group after the workout on Instagram and use the hashtag #trainingforlife.

MOVEMENT SNACKS

B Y THIS POINT, YOU can see all I really want people to do is start to think about the benefits of moving. To this day, the benefits of simply walking still blow my mind away. Walking has the potential to strengthen your heart, your muscles, bones, and improve health factors such as keeping triglycerides lower, and improve blood circulation. More often than not, a good walk can improve your mood too. Often times, walking is a perfect "Movement Snack," which is essentially a small bout of exercise done for one to five minutes that contracts or lengthens a muscle. This can involve doing some sort of exercise like walking or passive stretch anytime during the day, even multiple times per day.

Back in high school, we got a new gym teacher. I remember one of the first things I noticed about him was that he couldn't sit still. Once he stood up, I saw why: he was sitting on a Swiss ball. If you aren't sure what a Swiss ball is, imagine a bigger version of a beach ball that is designed for people to work out with. I asked him why he was sitting on it instead of chair and he said that "it beats sitting in a chair because it keeps my midsection engaged, which is good for the abs."

If you recall, abs are part of the core we talked about in the Longevity chapter, and by sitting on the Swiss ball, my teacher was "strengthening" his core. Now being a soccer player at the time, if you tell me that something is good for my core, I am going to give it a try. It wasn't long after that I found myself in a store buying a Swiss ball. Excited about my new piece of fitness equipment, I blew up my new purple Swiss ball, put it in my room, and decided that anytime I played video games I would sit on it instead of a chair or my bed. Then, something interesting happened.

My first movement snack

One day, between bouts of games, I rolled on the ball so that my feet were anchored to the ground and my upper back was on the ball. I started doing some crunches—no set number; I just did them until my next game started. Before I knew it, I was doing a movement snack.

After a few weeks of doing crunches, I would eventually hop on the floor between games and do pushups. I didn't really count sets or repetitions. Some days, I probably did three sets of fifteen to twenty sit ups and one set of twenty or so pushups. Other days, two sets of thirty crunches and five sets of twelve pushups. Sometimes it was just crunches or pushups. To some degree, one of my first programs I was consistent with outside of playing sports was doing either crunches or push-ups every ten to fifteen minutes, depending on the video game length. These Movement Snacks could potentially be the reason working out is now a habit I no longer need motivation for (more on that in a later chapter).

Less is more

I once had a client who was ready to change her life. At the time, I was doing intro sessions for new members. She was pumped to start her fitness journey and eager to do what it took to make some changes. I communicated that starting with two to three sessions a week was a good start. Instead, she went ALL IN and decided to do three to four group sessions each week: swimming for who knows how long and doing yoga and mobility classes on "off" days. At first thought, it was quite impressive. Being a younger coach, I thought to myself, "This is someone who is going to turn her life around fast!"

I was wrong. She only lasted two weeks (she hit the cliff), which bums me out until this day. She bit off more than she can chew. You often hear these incredible stories about how X and Y person made all these sacrifices and lost this crazy amount of weight in a short period of time. These anecdotes are extremely impressive and motivating but not realistic for everyone. We aren't all wired that way. Most of us will start with great intentions of making positive changes but then quickly fall off the wagon. Why? Too many of us look at lifestyle changes as pass or fail: "Oh I couldn't make it to the gym today; I'll try again tomorrow." Tomorrow comes... "That person responded to me on Tinder. Can't wait for my date tonight, I'll go to the gym tomorrow"... and then the next day your friend asks you to go out to the movies. And it just goes on and on. Speaking of the movies, they did a pretty cool thing actually (in theatres); during the previews they had a video on how you could use the new chairs to do crunches. Fitness professionals probably cringed because they did this while eating a bag of popcorn claiming it burns the calories you are eating. But what I appreciated was that they were showing—should I say it?—a movement snack.

How many snacks can I have?

So how do we restructure how we think about moving consistently day to day? Let us start with general guidelines that are recommended for physical activity. The Centers for Disease and Control and Prevention (CDC) recommends that we need about 150-300 minutes of moderate activity or seventy-five minutes of vigorous activity, daily. This seems to be the time frame where adults can get the most health benefits, whether that is doing something aerobic like running, brisk walking or muscle-building, such as pushups and sit-ups. These benefits go far beyond what you see in the mirror. Even though I occasionally like to flex my arm in the mirror, I know what is happening on the inside is going to pay off in the long run and keep my body—and your body—more resilient.

What is moderate or vigorous is relative. Working harder for half the time seems like a nice trade-off, but I am going to put my focus on that 150-minute recommendation. If you divide 150 by seven (for each day of the week), you get around twenty-one minutes. Now take that number and feel free to break it into chunks throughout the day. You can easily do three seven-minute bouts of movement, or five four-minute bouts. When you look and think of it that way, it doesn't seem so scary. Some of you might have even read the twenty-minute time frame and thought, *Oh, I can do that.*

All you need to do for a short period of time is either contract or lengthen some sort of muscles with movements that look like exercise and accumulate roughly 150 minutes throughout your week. If you like music, the average song is about four minutes long, so you just need to move for five songs a day! Put on a tune you like and just do anything. This is applicable to anyone who is busy, anyone who is just looking to get started, and those that could use more energy throughout their day. Honestly, we all could use more movement snacks. Even if it's jogging up and down stairs for three minutes, you are pushing the needle forward towards a healthier lifestyle.

Just start

You don't need to be in a certain spot in your life to achieve fitness—you just need to do something. My fitness journey started by sitting on an unstable ball for a bit, which then led to sit-ups, and then pushups, and eventually using some of the weights collecting dust in my basement. These small habits will build on themselves and bring you to what is sustainable for you. For me, that's five to six days a week in a gym. For others, it's three days a week in a gym and two days playing sports. Maybe, it's the weekend hike and yoga on Mondays and two home workouts throughout the week. When it comes to training for life, there is no perfect plan, only sustainability. Find something you can sustain for many years and you will reap the benefits. It doesn't need to be with an all-in mentality all the time. Now please excuse me while I go move around a little bit. I need a snack.

READER EXERCISE 4: Party Snack

We learned about movement snacks, so your next task is to play a song of your choice and you are going to rotate through the small circuit outlined below. Do as many rounds as possible (AMRAP) for the duration of your favourite song:
- 8 jumping jacks or side-step jacks (no jumping)
- 8 sit-to-stands from a chair or couch
- 8 shoulder taps from the top of a pushup, or with your hands on an elevated surface (couch or chair)

Record your circuit and post it on Instagram using the hashtag #trainingforlife.

MOTIVATION–DISCIPLINE–HABIT

MOTIVATION, DISCIPLINE, AND HABIT. I do not see any of these as equal and here's why. For the most part, when you talk to people about making changes in their personal lives, they often say that they aren't motivated. That brings up the question: What is motivation? It is a burst of desire to act upon something. Have you ever watched something like a boxing movie, and right after you feel like you want to start boxing? All of a sudden you get this rush to learn how to train and learn the art of boxing. Wait one week or so and that desire to be a boxer might or might not be there anymore—in my eyes, that's motivation.

Motivation is a temporary feeling that might help one start, and that's exactly what I want to focus on: how to start. I like to think everyone is motivated to get strong, to get rich, to do XYZ, but so many times people fail over and over. How can we get you from just being motivated to being disciplined? In order to be disciplined in something, you need motivation. In order to make something a habit, you need consistent discipline. This is a cycle we need to go through to make life changes that can benefit us.

When I was about seven or eight, I had a terrible habit of forgetting to brush my teeth. Mama was not impressed. Looking back now, I wasn't really motivated to do it. Why would I? My mouth didn't hurt, I didn't feel like my breath smelled bad, and I was probably more concerned about my Nintendo 64 than brushing my teeth. It got to the point where my mother had to put up signs around the house for me to remember to get the job done. So, what changed?

Finding a why

One day, the dentist who found a cavity in my mouth asked me about my brushing habits. My mom didn't hesitate to tell her, and never in my life has someone else cared so much about my teeth. The dentist was straight up giving me so much crap and warned me about what was going to happen my teeth if I didn't start taking care of them. Then she whipped out pictures of people who neglected their teeth and told me how lucky I was that my teeth weren't crooked and that no girl would ever want to kiss me, and my smile was going to be ugly. Some people might say that this dentist was harsh, but not in my eyes. This was exactly what I needed to hear. I could not begin to fathom the idea of no one wanting to kiss me! I also understood what she meant because I have had people with smoke breath hug me and kiss me on the cheek and I hated it. The dentist gave me the motivation and presented me the "why" behind the importance of oral hygiene.

Having a "why" attached to your motivation is much more likely to not only get you started but keep you on track towards your goals. This helps create discipline. Discipline in simple terms is the ability to pull yourself to doing what you need to do to achieve your goals. I would lay down, get all comfortable and about to sleep. Then the thought would pop up, *Oh man, I forgot to brush my teeth but I am so comfortable. Do I really want another cavity? Do I want to lose my teeth? What if I get to kiss my crush tomorrow?* Those were my whys, and they sure worked to get me up and out of my comfy bed to brush my teeth. That's discipline.

This is exactly what happens with fitness too. We get home from work and start to settle in, we get comfortable, and the thought of doing any physical activity is exhausting. The people who can silence that voice or push through it and go complete the task have discipline.

Then this interesting thing eventually starts to happen. Eventually, you don't really even think about it anymore, before bed, you just end up in the washroom over your sink, brushing and flossing your teeth. I even have one of those Waterpiks now just for fun; love them. They have these settings that can increase the pressure and I like to use it to spray Sam. I can wake up, do my day, and go to bed... and somewhere in there I have taken care of my oral hygiene without using too much brain power. That, folks, is habit. Habit is just part of your being; you don't have to think about it. This is the goal.

Pick a goal that resonates with you. If it's to become more fit and healthy, then ask yourself why. I have heard some say they want to dance at their daughter's wedding and they don't even have a child yet, but that is what keeps them going every day. I find a lot of times the why is much bigger than yourself. Maybe your initial "why" isn't for you but using it will directly benefit you and you will then love and enjoy the process. Your "why" WILL be your motivation, and you will never need to search for that again. Eventually, you will just be disciplined enough to act and stay consistent, which will finally just turn into a habit, and it will be part of who you are.

READER EXERCISE 5: Your Why

For this reader exercise, grab a pen or pencil and a small piece of paper or use the notes app on your phone. Write down a couple of big reasons why fitness and health are important to you. Try to find something that you put a lot of value in. Next time you feel like you don't want to do something that could push the needle of fitness and health forward, refer back to what you wrote.

If you are comfortable sharing your "why," then post it on Instagram and use the hashtag #trainingforlife.

GETTING LOVED ONES MOVING

FOLLOWING UP ON THE last chapter, everyone is going to land under some category on a different spectrum on where they are in regard to motivation, discipline, and habit for each aspect of their life, and that is completely okay. The fact that you are reading this might mean there is already an interest in bettering yourself. Maybe you already consider yourself fit, healthy, and happy; perhaps maybe this is the guide that will kickstart it for you; or maybe you are a loved one who had this book referred to them to get you motivated to start your journey.

It seems to be very human to want to share great things with others. I often see people around me telling me how they are convincing their friends to try X diet or X gym and that it has changed their personal lives. I often question what their approach is. I know it can be difficult to get some people to make habit changes as they might live a completely different lifestyle than you. To add to that, how you approach loved ones can make or break the message you are trying to get across.

I have convinced many people near and dear to my heart to start to MOVE and just THINK about what is means to eat better. Just move and think, not necessarily join a gym, or go on a crazy fad diet. The best part is at some point, they eventually ask questions like "Hey, what do you think about running for this long?" and "How much rice should I have per meal?" When I start to hear those questions, I get fired up because they are now considering moving and food quantity. This is a much better, more realistic way to convince someone to start to take care of their body, versus throwing them in the deep end and asking them to join you five days a week and eat chicken and broccoli four to five times a day.

Time and time again, I have seen success with people who ease into things through movement snacks or making the conscious decision to put a little more vegetables on their plate. I'll be the first one to tell you that I haven't always had the perfect approach to getting people I care about to start. But looking back now, I got them all to start, whether it took a couple of months or a couple of years. Sometimes the message was rough, and sometimes it was sprinkled in conversation as a trick.

My parents are a good example of people it took me a couple of years to convince. My dad lifted weights way before I was born. In fact, he bought a weight set that I was lucky enough to have as my first home gym. I knew he was always into building some muscle, staying healthy, and busting his sleeves. He has had some unfortunate events that pushed training off at times. He was hurting his back, he had appendicitis, surgeries, and some other life obstacles that prevented him from getting after it in the gym short term. But to his benefit, he also told me a phrase that I remember until this day, "The squeaky wheel gets the grease."

After a while, I realized I just needed to be his "squeaky wheel." I talk about the benefits of lifting weights, moving, and studies on all things fitness and health related often around him. Being his only son, he had no choice but to listen, and I am very good at repeating myself (squeaky wheel). I eventually got him to work with me one on one! This was fun; he would come into the gym twice a week for a short while, and I got him to lift some weights and occasionally get his heart rate up. Life happened once again, so that had to stop for a bit. So now what? What can I do?

After a couple of months, I wanted to get my dad to start again. I realized he was busy and generally tired when he got home, which is understandable when your workday averages ten to twelve hours. I also know that exercising doesn't need to last an hour. I knew he climbed up and down stairs all day long, so what could I do to help him? I called him up excited and said, "I have an idea!" He laughed on the other end and said,

"What is it?" I said, "You're a busy guy, you work long hours, BUT there is this one lift a day program. It's simple: you just pick a lift and do… "

I continued to explain the routine, then wrote down everything for him. I printed and posted it on the wall of his home gym for him to follow along. The program was simple, and I knew he had experience with these movements. He did back squats on Monday, bent over rows on Tuesday, Romanian deadlifts on Thursday, and Arnold Press on Saturdays. If others wish to try, I suggest you start with an empty barbell and light dumbbells (five to fifteen pounds, depending on your experience) and build on it over time slowly. A rule of thumb that is good to follow is to add up to ten pounds for lower body movements per week and up to five pounds on upper body movements per week. The program looked like so:

Week 1: 7 sets of 5 reps of each movement
Week 2: 6 sets of 3 reps of each movement
Week 3: 1 set of 5, 1 set of 3, and 1 final set of 2 reps of each movement
Week 4: 4 sets of 12 reps of each movement

When done correctly, Week 1 is a very tough workout! The goal isn't necessarily to hold the same weight across all the sets (if you are a beginner, I would keep the weight the same), but use the first few sets to warm up. Maybe sets four and five are tough, and then you can back off the weight for the final two sets. Let's look below and assume this person is squatting and has a 280-pound back squat for two reps. The seven sets might look like this:

Set 1: 135 x 5   Set 5: 230 x 5
Set 2: 165 x 5   Set 6: 205 x 5
Set 3: 185 x 5   Set 7: 205 x 5
Set 4: 205 x 5

Week 2 has pretty much half the volume with a total of eighteen reps. This means you can push the loads a little bit more and get heavier with your weights. In the Week 1 example, we did 230 pounds for a set of five reps as the heavy set. For Week 2, add ten to twenty pounds to that and use that weight for your sets of three. For this layout, I would suggest to warm up, build with the first two to three sets, and then hold the same heavy weight for three to four sets.

Set 1: 185 x 3   Set 4: 250 x 3
Set 2: 215 x 3   Set 5: 250 x 3
Set 3: 235 x 3   Set 6: 250 x 3

Week 3 is a fun one. This is one set of five reps, one set of three reps, and one set of two reps. We are essentially warming up, and then across these three sets building up to a challenging two reps for the day.

Set 1: 235 x 5
Set 2: 250 x 3
Set 3: 270 x 2

On Week 4, we de-load the weight and move much slower through each rep. This is a nice break from the heavier weeks to allow your body to recover with four sets of twelve reps and prepare itself for the next month's progression, which hopefully means you can start to add a little bit of load OR the same load until it feels easier. I have to give credit to Coach Dan John who popularized this program back in 2004. The only difference from the original program is that he tells people to take the fourth week off, but I am not asking my dad to max out or push the weights till his eyes pop out. I simply want him to move some external load in a reasonable time frame, with a simple approach, for as much of the calendar year as possible.

With this program my dad went from not lifting any weights to now lifting at least four times per week! That's a big win in my book. Strength is very important to attain and sustain, especially as you get older. Even better, in between sets my dad started doing some exercises for smaller muscle groups, without me even prescribing it—an even bigger win.

How did I do it? I've been consistently sprinkling in the benefits, ideas, and recommendations of fitness for more than eight years in the moments we are together, usually through conversation. The best time to start was yesterday, the next best time to start is today, but sometimes it's also better late than never. So, to my fitness friends, start being the squeaky wheel. Not the loud obnoxious kind, but the kind that the driver can turn the music up to once in a while and pretend nothing is wrong. Eventually, they need to grease the wheel. If they decide to change the tire… well, I got nothing for you there.

READER EXERCISE 6: Squeaky Wheel

For this task, see if you can be a squeaky wheel to someone you care about. You don't have to be annoying. If they're motivated to move, have them go on a walk with you or join you for a stretch. Depending on how well you know the person, maybe even sign up for a short event together like a five-kilometre run or walk. These small steps can help make big differences in peoples' lives. It might just be what they were waiting for.

Post a picture of you and the friend you're being a squeaky wheel to! Go on Instagram and use the hashtag #trainingforlife.

STRESS

What is stress?

STRESS COMES IN MANY forms, and it's something every human will experience regardless of who you are, what you do, or how you grew up. Stress relates to everyday life mentally, and it also relates to physical training. For starters, let's focus on the type of stress you might deal with on a regular basis. There's something called "eustress," which is typically associated with things we perceive as positive, such as getting a promotion at work, completing a challenging task, or even the joy from riding a roller coaster.

"Distress" is typically associated with something that is negative. This is usually what we think about when we use the term "stress." When it comes to training for life, I like to think it is more than what you just physically do but how you manage what is going on in between the ears, which is usually easier said than done. So many factors affect us on a daily basis and everyone's experience is unique. We don't know the burdens people carry in their personal lives. Some of us may be experiencing mental health challenges. Maybe a loved one has passed away, or perhaps you've had a life-changing experience that is tough to deal with. These are all examples of major stressors. Then there are also minor, smaller stress that don't seem as important in the day to day, but with time they can add up. These are the small decisions you need to make on a regular basis. Small stressors can affect everyday life.

Effects of stress

The effects of stress can be put into two categories: acute stress and chronic stress. Think of acute stress as a short-term moment where you feel like your heart is beating fast, you need to take a big deep breath, and maybe even feel the butterflies in your stomach. For some, this happens when you are about to go in front of a room to put on a presentation or maybe you are about to do your first ever local five-kilometre race.

Chronic stress is long term. This is when you are in an environment or have developed a lifestyle that is constantly putting stress on the body and can eventually trigger mental or physical health issues. Some examples are depression, cardiovascular disease, or diabetes.

Stress can affect us all in different ways. One common thing we know is that if there is a constant imbalance of stress, it can make some changes to our bodies. It can increase your heart rate, it can raise your blood pressure, make it more challenging to sleep etc... This can make it really difficult to find an optimal level of health, which is why it is important to learn to manage stress.

Identifying types of stress

One thing that is important to understand is that what is considered a big or small stressor is all relative to the person who is experiencing it. When people come to me and we discuss their training goals, I usually focus on three things first. How are they sleeping? How are they eating? How is their stress management? Notice that we don't talk about their training program. Those three factors, if not taken seriously, will put too much strain on the mind and body. The training results will take longer to achieve and also may not be achieved at all since the body may struggle to find balance.

How to manage stress

I have heard many different approaches when it comes to managing stress, and what's key is to find what works best for you. First, I think it comes down to your personal attitude. I believe your attitude is one of the first things you must change to manage your stress. If you see every situation as negative one and put blame on outside factors for things that happen in your life, then you are constantly blaming things that are outside of your control. I find when people take ownership and responsibility for their actions, there is a shift in their attitude and they start to enjoy finding solutions to problems. To add to that, we must deal with our issues or problems as they occur. If you leave something and try to deal with it later, then there are good chances it will eventually stress you out. You need to attack anything you are dealing with right away.

Dealing with it right away might include those tough conversations, typing up that email, finding a solution that your team can appreciate. Through any moment in life where I felt stressed, taking action has always made it feel better. The initial step is the hardest one to take, but when the ball starts rolling, this weight gets lifted off of your shoulders.

Now, something I mentioned earlier is blaming things out of your control. I find this is the most common thing we, as people, do. There are so many things that are out of our control that add stressors to our life. Let's discuss one element that none of us can control: the weather. In 2016, I had the opportunity to visit Iceland (highly recommended) and I remember hiking with some friends through one of the national parks. I kid you not, within about a two- to three-hour window, it went from warm to chilly to hot to chilly to warm again. At first, I thought it was just me, but all my friends noticed it too. Luckily, we had been warned about Iceland's weather, so I was prepared. I pack an extra sweater and a winter jacket. There is a saying: There is no bad weather only bad clothing.

We are so good at knowing that we cannot control the weather so we plan for it. We focus on the things we can control, so that if it decides to rain on us, the umbrellas are ready and we are happy. If we didn't, well then, we are cold, wet, and upset that it's raining.

Stress and training

So, what does stress have to do with training? Everything really, as training in itself is a stressor. So why do people love to exercise? Besides its long-term effects, it has short-term effects too and releases the "feel good" chemicals from our brains called endorphins. These act as a natural painkiller and tends to put people at ease afterwards. This is why people also love to do meditation, massage therapy, or even focused deep breathing: it can cause your body to produce the same hormones.

Physical movement is a stress release, whether it is playing a sport, running, lifting weights, chopping wood, doing yoga, or anything that involves using our bodies and feeling present. When you are working out, it is really hard to focus on executing a squat while trying to plan dinner. Working out requires you to have full focus on what you are doing. This is why I think lifting weights or doing circuit training is like meditation in itself because it forces you to stay in the moment and concentrate on your movement and breathing. If you get distracted, you have to bring your attention back to what you are doing so you can be effective with the task at hand.

Besides moving, working out will also improve other areas of your life, like lowering stress, which in turn can help with your sleep. If you have quality sleep and recover better, this has shown to help boost mood, cognitive function, and improve your overall performance, whether in the gym or office. One thing I have observed is that a lot of highly successful people always make time to take care of their bodies first, which I think keeps stress levels lower overall. Since they are getting quality sleep and keeping their body moving, this makes them more effective day to day.

So how do we control our stress better? You want to remove any unnecessary things from your life that brings you stress, focus on what you can control, and USE your body! There's just something about doing squats and burpees that makes you feel good—sometimes.

READER EXERCISE 7: 5x5 Rule

For this task I want us all to embrace the 5x5 rule when it comes to handling stress. It takes time to get good at. The 5x5 rule is this: If it isn't going to matter in five years, then don't spend more than five minutes thinking about it. That's it. The next time you feel stressed, spend five minutes thinking about what is stressing you out, why. etc. If it is going to matter, then you need to take action and address it. If it is not, then you need to let it go.

Let us know how the 5x5 method worked for you on Instagram. Use the hashtag #trainingforlife.

SLEEP

LOVE SLEEP! MANY PEOPLE are often looking for more energy, better mood, and just looking to feel awesome—the answer is better sleep. I am often shocked at how sleep is the first thing we are willing to sacrifice in order to get things done. It honestly makes no sense to me. Sleep is the most effective recovery tool we as humans have and most likely ever will have. Yet, as a whole, our society is sleep deprived. Even worse, some people say they don't have time to sleep when often times they are on their smartphone or watching TV for two to three hours before getting shut-eye (heads up: that's making your sleep quality worse).

Since my younger days, I have always preferred to go to bed early. I remember when my mother graduated me from going to bed from 8:30 to 9; I thought it was the coolest thing ever only to realize now that it was still early. But if there is one habit I am thankful for, it's that she taught me to hit the sheets at a consistent time. Once I hit college, that's when I really noticed how tired everyone was. The only time I would stay up late was when I was talking until 3 to 4 a.m. with my partner Sam (okay, maybe giving up sleep is worth love), but besides that, I never saw the point. I would wake up for exams and hear things like, "I stayed up until 2 to 3 a.m. studying for this exam," only for them to fail the exam. Now you lost sleep and you failed. Good job.

Side note: There is nothing wrong with staying up past your normal bedtime SOMETIMES… but if it is affecting your health and your lifestyle then it's important to take note.

What happens to us when we don't sleep enough?

Let's start with your professional life. It is going to make your productivity worse as compared to a restful night of sleep, mainly because it has shown that people who lack sleep are not thinking as sharp and have the increased potential to making poor decisions. For this reason alone, I really feel for our emergency services, nurses, doctors, etc., because they are usually asked to do very important jobs while under extreme fatigue.

Along with that, lack of sleep affects our physical health, our chances of dealing with cardiovascular diseases, diabetes, and obesity, and immunodeficiency start to increase, which is not good. These issues make life much more challenging and take away from what can be and should be an enjoyable experience. This can all start to improve if we take sleep just a bit more seriously.

Fixing sleep

So how do we make sleep more effective when we do get time? I have learned more and more and put lots into practice. Lots of trial and error to see what works the best. I'll give you arguably the most important one right now… consistency. Pick a bedtime, pick a wake-up time, and try and do that as often as possible to build a proper circadian rhythm in your body. What is a circadian rhythm? It's a natural internal clock that regulates our sleep–wake cycle. Aim to do this seven days a week.

Now, I should add that we should be getting at the very least seven hours of sleep, eight is ideal according to the National Health Services (NHS). Look at someone like Usain Bolt, the first man to win six gold medals in the sport of sprinting at the Summer Olympic Games. He sleeps about eight to ten hours a night to rest and recover from his training. According to Fatigue Science, which is a sleep-performance software company, football players reduce their forty-yard dash by 0.1 seconds when they sleep more. This may not seem like much time, but in high-level performance sports, 0.1 seconds is the different between a silver or a gold, a touch down or a fumble.

I do wish it was as easy as pick a bedtime and a wake time to get a full rest. Did you know horses only need to sleep about three hours? Imagine going to bed at 12 a.m. and waking up at 3 a.m. fully rested. That would be pretty awesome, but we aren't horses so please don't do that. I only bring this up because some folks claim they are work horses, that they have barely slept all week, and they are "grinding," but they move and think slower than molasses. So, when choosing a sleep–wake routine, please aim for something between seven to nine hours.

Next up: your environment. You want your room and your bed to be a place your body and mind can feel at rest when it is time to do so. Start with making sure you invest in a comfortable bed—you spend at least one-third of your life on your mattress; it is very well worth the investment. Nowadays, you can get a pretty comfortable mattress for a decent price. Once you have the mattress set, it has been shown to help if you have a cooler room before going to bed. It is beneficial to sleep in a temperature that is cooler because, first, how much nicer do those sheets feel when you are all snuggled up? And second, sleeping in a cooler room will help drop our body temperature, which then increases melatonin production. Melatonin is a hormone that gets released to help us with the sleep–wake cycle.

Having good melatonin production is important for us to fall asleep and keep us asleep. There are many things that can mess with melatonin production, which brings me to another tip to improve sleep: put away screens such as TVs, phones, tablets and, if possible, dim the lights in your house. There are some recommendations to turn all screens off at least one hour before bed. For some people, this can be extremely difficult, especially if you like to look at your phone for two to three hours while in bed. But you want to avoid this! Screen time before bed has shown to make falling asleep harder and makes it challenging to stay in a deep sleep due to the psychological stimulation you get from watching cat videos on Instagram.

How do you fill that hour before bed? Create a bedtime routine. This can be unique to you but do something that helps you relax. I'll share my routine as a small example:

1. Stage your house for the morning (get clothes ready, food, pack bags etc.).
2. Make and enjoy a nighttime snack (I like yogurt with some casein protein).
3. Brush my teeth and floss.
4. Take a hot shower.
5. Play tug of war with my puppy until we are both done.
6. Go out like a light.

Keep it simple

Notice how it's nothing fancy, but it is something I do on a regular basis before bed. Some people like to stretch or do mindful breathing, and all of that is awesome. For me, it's the process I follow which allows me to clear my mind, and that is ultimately the goal.

As you can see, there are a couple of things you can get to work on right away. And I want to mention just one more before I close off this chapter: when to eliminate caffeine. Oftentimes when we think of caffeine, we think of coffee. But there is also caffeine in some teas, some carbonated drinks, energy drinks, and even chocolate.

Ultimately, caffeine is a stimulant for the brain. It stays in our system a little longer than most people think, and this can affect your ability to fall asleep and have a restful night. According to the Sleep Foundation, it is recommended to avoid consuming caffeine within six hours of your desired bedtime. If you find that is not enough and still struggle to fall asleep, a lot of specialists in the nutritional world recommend to cut out caffeine a bit earlier and experiment to find a time frame that works for you. This can depend on different factors but the key is to try and keep track of how you slept before and after you eliminated the caffeine.

Now you have some actionable items on your list to improve the time you spend with your eyelids closed. Start with one or two and slowly layer more and more on over time to truly make this a habit. Sleep well.

READER EXERCISE 8: Sleep Plan

It is time to improve your sleep! For this next task, what I'd like you to do is start with developing a plan for your sleep routine. To review, some things you want to consider are a consistent bedtime and wake up time, a relaxing and comfortable environment, a good routine, and seven-plus hours of sleep per night. Start with building consistency by choosing a bedtime and a wake time. This will be hard at first, but I promise you can put the phone down! Next, write a small routine you want to do before shut-eye. Start there and let's see how it goes!

Post your bedtime routine to Instagram and use the hashtag #trainingforlife.

DIET

WHEN IT COMES TO talking about diet and how people should be eating, I would say there is a mass confusion on what is the optimum way to eat. When it comes to food, there is a social, emotional, and geographical impact, whether that is religion or what food you have access to. You might have heard of some common diets by now such as the Mediterranean diet, paleo, intermittent fasting, keto, blood type, vegan, Atkins®, the Zone diet®. I could go on and on! You will hear different people claim one to be optimal and the "best" one for you or my personal favourite: "This is how we are supposed to eat."

It's no wonder people have no idea what information is right and wrong. It creates such frustration for those who truly just want to find a healthy balance in their life when it comes to food. Food is the one thing you need from the moment you are born to the moment you die. It is what fuels you and gives you energy. Yet, no one has ever really been taught how to properly eat, which inevitably has created some societies that are now, on average, overweight. I, too, have been pulled into trying some of these diets. The last one taught me lots of good lessons on how to approach food.

I was skimming through the wonderful world of YouTube and watching some of my favourite athletes' vlogs. I came across a couple of them mentioning how they started to do intermittent fasting. It raised a few red flags, but I was intrigued. Rich Froning and Josh Bridges both have knee pain from overuse, which they mentioned was getting better due to following this diet. They claimed their testosterone went up, and both just over felt much better and more energized for their training. I thought to myself, *My left knee is not feeling great these days. I train similarly to these two people I just watched, and personally, I don't think there is anything wrong with me raising my testosterone.*

When you hear these experiences from others, it makes you question if it can work for you. Who doesn't want to feel healthy and perform well day to day? And not just performance in the gym, I am talking about everyday life as well. Now, just to explain what intermittent fasting is, it is essentially a diet where you have a set period of time where you do not eat food, and a set period of time where you do eat, which is called a "feeding window." There are different fasting time frames people play with, but the most common one is sixteen hours of no eating followed by an eight-hour feeding window. Most people who do this usually stop eating around 9 p.m. at night and won't start until 1 p.m. the next day.

People usually use intermittent fasting as a way to lose weight because when you limit eating for a period of the day, it typically puts you in a caloric deficit (less calories than your body utilizes that day). So, it can be quite effective, but only if the person doesn't use the feeding window as an opportunity to binge. Losing weight wasn't my goal though. So, I downloaded a calorie tracker right away to make sure I was eating enough calories to continue to gain weight (caloric surplus), as I still wanted to add muscle mass and strength during this period. I wanted to do intermittent fasting because of the benefits these particular athletes were claiming. You can say I got suckered into the hype.

Weeks in, I noticed improvements in everything that I wanted. I was gaining weight, I was sleeping better, my body was feeling like a rock star, but I still had questions. I had questions because my approach to nutrition had completely changed. Was it the intermittent fasting? Or was it the fact that I was now more aware of what was going into my body?

I had a call with a very good friend who coaches people in nutrition and we discussed my experience. We talked about how I was approaching this and how I was seeing results. My friend being who he is, was super-awesome and ready to give me scientific information. We concluded that the diet that I was on, followed by my goals, actually forced me to drink more water and be more mindful when I eat. I started to eat way more vegetables and whole foods in general. I became much better at preparing my meals and, for the first time, actually getting in enough calories to support my activity levels. As soon as we finished up that phone call, I realized that intermittent fasting in itself was not magical, but it gave me habits I didn't have previously. I told myself I was going back eating at whatever time I wanted, but not changing what I was now eating. I can honestly tell you I felt the exact same as when intermittent fasting.

So why did it technically work for me in the first place? I was honestly concerned about not getting enough calories and nutrients to support my lifestyle. This forced me to prepare my meals better to make sure any time I put something in my mouth it was going to fuel me properly. Ultimately, everyone has needs that are unique to them as individuals. Intermittent fasting was not going to be a sustainable approach for me, but it did teach me some lessons.

Calories matter for weight gain and loss

Another thing stood out too: calories in, calories out does work. In fact, when it comes strictly to weight loss, calories matter most. Mark Haub, a professor of human nutrition at Kansas State University experimented with a "Twinkie diet" for ten weeks and lost twenty-seven pounds. This diet was two thirds of junk food, but he would also have a protein shake, have some vegetables and took a multivitamin. He limited himself to 1,800 calories daily to put him in a caloric deficit. Haub wouldn't recommend this diet, but it proves a point that energy balance is what truly matters when it comes to weight loss or weight gain. In fact, we can't even blame our metabolism any more as a study published in the *Science Journal* has shown our total daily energy expenditure is stable between the ages of twenty to sixty. Even when we hit sixty years old, it slows down by only 0.7 per cent per year. So why do we gain weight during those years? We are simply moving less and less.

In the nutrition world, there are claims about so many factors as to why people cannot lose body fat, which seem to go against the concept of calories in, calories out. Acclaimed professionals say that its either hormones or… Nope, wait; it's the sugar… Wait, nope; it's definitely the carbs. I can tell you right now that I have eaten cereal and lost weight and eaten cereal and gained weight. It comes down to if you are consuming more calories than you expend or vice versa, depending on your goals. Any registered dietitian will likely tell you that the most effective way to lose weight is to be in a caloric deficit and to gain weight, a caloric surplus. This has been proven over a few studies that show intermittent energy restriction and daily energy restriction have comparable numbers when it comes to weight loss. Energy restriction is another way of saying caloric deficit, which is where we typically lose weight/ body fat.

The problem with certain foods such as cereals or cookies is that they are extremely calorically dense and don't carry much nutritional value compared to fruits and vegetables. They also are not very filling. This means you will probably eat more or become hungrier faster when consuming processed foods. Tracking your food to a degree is useful at first, so you can keep an eye on how much you are truly putting in your body.

Trust me: I wish a tablespoon of peanut butter was a tall, little mountain resting on my spoon—but it's not. That doesn't mean I can't enjoy peanut butter; I just need to control my portion. When food is processed, a lot of the nutrients in the food are removed. Some of these nutrients are fibre, which produce satiety (the feeling of being full). Proteins (chicken, beef etc.) and whole plant foods (broccoli, spinach, etc.) are very satiating and lay a solid foundation for any diet.

Who to listen to

I'll be the first to admit that I don't envy anyone who works in nutrition because of the stuff they hear and need to deal with, like having all the nutrition gurus running around and demonizing ways of eating. When I tried intermittent fasting, someone made a funny comment to me: "Are the one hundred calories you eat different at 8:59 p.m. then then are at 9:01 p.m.?" No. No, they are not.

So how should I eat? Look, I am not here to prescribe a plan to anyone. I think some good rules to follow are eat a variety of fruits and veggies, get adequate amounts of animal protein (enough to support your lifestyle), drink a good amount of water per day, and get some good sleep.

Another thing which I think will be of value to you is understanding who NOT to listen to when it comes to nutritional information. Here are some red flags to look out for:

- anyone who speaks in absolutes
- anyone who demonizes specific foods or food groups
- anyone who is selling a product to enhance your diet
- people who say, "If you eat like me, you'll look like me"
- anyone who isn't a registered dietitian

Registered dietitians are properly trained to give out information that is evidence-based and can truly provide you with a personalized plan. A nutritionist is not typically held accountable by a regulatory college. That being said, I have personally encountered incredible, logical, very smart nutritionists who do the same effective work as a registered dietitian, BUT be careful and search for those red flags. As soon as you start to sense a bias in nutritional information, I would immediately start asking questions and/or get a second opinion.

If you can start to weed out the good information from the bad, that can be a huge benefit both physically and mentally when it comes to nutrition. It truly is a small journey in itself when it comes to understanding how to eat according to you and figuring out the most effective ways to fuel and enjoy food in your day-to-day life.

READER EXERCISE 9: Food Log

It is safe to say that the majority of us love food! With this exercise, I want to present a challenge. For the next seven days, write down everything you eat and drink! (Be honest!) After the seven days, look at your food log and see where you can make improvements.

Post your food log to Instagram and use the hashtag #trainingforlife.

FIND WHAT WORKS

U P TO THIS POINT, we have talked about some extremely important topics that play a role into longevity and some good starting
steps or thoughts to improving ourselves. Let's imagine the shape of a
triangle right now: put sleep on one corner, nutrition on the opposite side,
and training on the remaining corner. A triangle is known as the strongest
shape because if you apply pressure on to one side, the force is equally distributed on the other two sides. I like to think of it like this: If I eat better,
then my sleep and my training are going to be better, and if I sleep better,
I am going to perform better, which keeps me more consistent to eating
the calories I need, since according to studies, poor sleepers tend to have
higher risk for obesity. Lastly, if I train well, my sleep quality will improve.
Personally, I feel like when you start to use your body more, you want to
give it the fuel it needs to have energy, which makes it easier to develop
better eating habits when you start to move.

I guess the question is: How should you move? If you recall to some
earlier chapters, I am a fan of people increasing their physical capacity through adding it in their daily lives, whether that is walking more,
or hiking, going out and playing a sport, as well as add those movement
snacks throughout your day so you can accumulate as much movement as
possible. Honestly, it can be anything that helps push the needle forward
of health and wellness, but I do always recommend finding a solid routine

for working out. Nowadays though, there is so much buzz, so many different things you can do. You have gyms styles for high intensity circuit training (HIIT), strength-only gyms, yoga, running clubs, conventional gyms, gymnastics, swimming… There is honestly so much. And that is the beauty of it.

I was fortunate enough to start in a fitness program called CrossFit® where the intent of the program is to include as many styles of training as possible in one program. You have the Olympic lifts such as the snatch and the clean and jerk, but also power-lifting, which includes the squat, bench press and deadlift. Another type of training included is gymnastics, which involves moving your bodyweight through space. And don't just think tumbling and handstand walks: pull-ups and pushups are considered gymnastics, too. In addition, we also do something called mono-structural work, which includes higher-repetition work like running, swimming, and biking. Those are the main three, but there is so much more.

It is super fun learning so many new skills at once and figuring out how to lift a barbell, kettlebell, or atlas stones. Equally fulfilling is learning how to master the muscle up, a movement where you execute a pull up on a pair of rings, do a big sit up to get the rings below your shoulders and then you press down (imagine getting out of the deep end of a pool). You start to really enjoy what your body can do and expressing your fitness in different ways. It's addicting because you didn't realize all the cool things the body is capable of doing.

Having a program with this kind of variety can give someone a lifetime of fitness. One thing I started to notice over the long haul, though, is that occasionally people start to gravitate towards one or the other a little more. Some people start to geek out about the barbell and want to become better at Olympic weightlifting. Others dabble into the endurance world and start to challenge themselves on how far they can run, whether it was a marathon or a 100 mile race. It is actually really cool to see because each style has its own world that you can dig into if it interests you. That's the important part of zeroing in on a workout or exercise style: Does it actually interest you?! The best thing about picking a style of training now is that there is so much variety. If you are someone who is looking for longevity, playing with different programs is okay! That being said, I recommend sticking with most programs for at least eight to twelve weeks, so you can reap the benefits of your efforts.

You often hear some trainers scoff at some forms of exercise, which starts to create a close-minded client. This takes away something a particular person might enjoy as a way to achieve fitness. As a coach myself, yes there are things to look out for, but for the most part, unless you are trying to squat on one leg, while on one of the big exercise balls and holding all your pets, I believe most movements have a place in the exercise world. I am looking more at things like running. Some say running is bad, but is it really? Some will say deadlifts are bad, but are they really? No. Running and deadlifting are perfectly safe, especially if a coach helps you progress in a safe manner.

At the end of the day, it comes down to what your personal goals are and how you want to achieve fitness that day, that month, and that year. Know that it's okay to change if that's what will keep you motivated long-term. If you have no clue where or how to start, then research might be key.

A simple trick when you are really at a crossroads for what to do is google "gyms around me" and take a few weeks to shop around. There is a bonus chapter at the end of the book that will give you some guidance on what you can get based on prices and experience. Once you have an idea of what you are looking for, search for free trials and free sessions/consultations. Look for a place that encourages you to move safely and has a plan to help you progress towards your fitness goals.

I personally have seen lots of success with the group model of training, because what inevitably happens is you become part of a community that wants to see you succeed. If you haven't shown up in a week or so, you might notice one day your classmates will start texting you, asking where you are. This kind of support can help get you back in the groove if you have had an off week or so.

You might not really know what you like until you try it. I do have to throw a wrench in the mix though. No matter what style you choose, there is one thing that is pretty key for longevity—and that, folks, is some sort of strength training. Whether you do it twice a week or four times a week usually depends on where your time is being spent.

READER EXERCISE 10: Jack of all Trades

For this chapter's exercise, I challenge you to try three different modes of exercise. This can be anything. Go drop in to a boxing gym, and the next day visit an Olympic weightlifting gym, yoga studio, etc. If you don't want to drop in to gyms (they usually have free trials), just try something different than what you are doing right now!

Post a picture of the gym you tried out on Instagram and give them some love! Use the hashtag #trainingforlife.

STRENGTH

What is considered strength?

STRENGTH CAN VARY AND mean one thing to one person and another to someone else. You can look at a parent carrying two kids at once and consider that strong. You can see the bulging bicep of a waste collector throwing the garbage in the truck and recognize that as strong. Perhaps you consider those who lift heavy weights strong; maybe it's a strongman athlete or a powerlifter. In my books, all these people are strong as strength is relative and it truly does depend on what their personal goals are in life, but also what life asks of them.

Now in sport, weight training, for the most part, is a staple. Usually, coaches keep what is in the weight room relative to the tasks the athlete will be completing depending on the domain they are in. Some movements are to increase power, others are to prevent injury, but all in all, they want resilient, stronger, and faster athletes. The person who doesn't play sports and just wants to feel good and be independent through life can and should also do the same thing, with just a different mindset and approach as it can provide lifelong benefits.

I once read a quote from Dr. John Rusin, a reputable trainer and physiotherapist who said, "Age is not a disability, so stop treating it like one." The reason I bring this up is because people tend to use their age as an excuse to not lift weights. We need to reframe our mindset here: As you age, you should be doing some form of resistance exercise (moving your-self or weights through space) at least two times a week for as long as your body allows. Weight training with a proper plan can help address some bone and joint limitations, such as arthritis, osteoporosis, muscle atrophy (loss of muscle), and many others. Retaining or gaining muscle mass has shown to help us live longer and be more independent. It helps us push off the nursing home and allows you to have a higher-quality life.

Age is just a number

I used to have a client; let's say her name is Sofia. She was in her fifties. Sofia was super eager to begin training and joined our gym to get some fitness on. At first, she wasn't very strong and had limited range of motion (more on range of motion coming up). Sofia joined with a family member who was much younger, moved well, and had some solid strength. Unfortunately, the younger one didn't stick around. Maybe Sofia needed to be a squeakier wheel. We used to program this exercise called a yoke carry, which is incredible for total body strength and work capacity.

A yoke is a piece of equipment that has a thick bar that sits on your shoulders with vertical metal poles that hold it up—kind of a square frame with the yoke bar (called a crossmember) horizontally on top. Usually, you drop the bar a couple of inches below your shoulders, so when you pick it up there are about four to six inches of space between the poles and the ground. Most people get pretty intimidated when they see a yoke for the first time, but Sofia was not scared of the yoke at all. In fact, she went under it and tried to stand up but couldn't. I recommended that we do something else and we did. She wasn't upset about it, but now she had a goal. She trained consistently two to three times per week for a few months before I decided to test yoke carries again.

I had just finished reviewing how I wanted everyone to approach the yoke. The safest way to pick it up and to drop it. I organized everyone into two groups. I remember asking Sofia if she wanted to do something else. She said, "No, I think I am going to try this." Boom! She picked it up easily and walked with it as if there was nothing on her back. I forgot to mention that the yoke on its own is 185 pounds! Which is ridiculously impressive for a five foot two woman weighing about 120 pounds. She made it look natural.

When Sofia completed the fifty-foot walk, she grabbed some ten-pound plates and placed one each of the four corners, bringing the weight up to 225 pounds. When she picked that yoke up with that much weight and walked it for another fifty feet, put it down, and smiled, I kid you not, I had a small tear in my eye. It was so cool watching someone who looked "fragile" develop and get stronger despite her age, which is often an excuse people use. She gained confidence and strength, which often offers more independence. And, most importantly, she put some years on her life.

Carry your way to strength

The yoke is a great test because you have to lift up a heavy weight and carry it a certain distance. I typically use fifty feet as a base when working with heavier weights. It is a great test of full body strength. Now, I am aware not everyone has access to a yoke but loaded carries such as the farmer's carry or bearhug carry in general have a similar carry-over (no pun intended). I love carries for developing strength because there is often a very fast learning curve.

In the world of fitness, it is quite popular to see exercise selections based around movements such as squats, presses, and pulls, which are essential and necessary to building well rounded strength. BUT—I believe we can all include more loaded carries and holds. The strongest people I have ever learned from have often said the same thing: Carry heavy things often. It might not be something you see often in a gym, but there are some simple ways to include it in your routine.

For a farmer's carry, grab a pair of dumbbells or kettlebells that you think would be challenging. Now farmers carry them for thirty seconds. Was it easy? Okay, now rest for sixty to ninety seconds and do the same thing but with heavier weights, say, five to ten pounds more. When you find it challenging to hold on for the thirty seconds, that is a good weight! You can do three to four sets and reap tons of benefits from that.

You can have a similar approach with movements like the bearhug, which is typically done with a sandbag. As you become more experienced with the types of loads you can manage, you can start to challenge yourself by doing max holds, or max distance! A fun test I personally like to do every once or twice a year, is see how heavy I can farmer's carry for fifty feet.

Train to sustain

When it comes to strength training for longevity, there are some key points to keep in mind. One is trying to reach a full range of motion to which your body currently allows. Don't just think of strength as how much you can lift, but in what range of motion you can lift it too. Another is loading your body accordingly, whether that is with carries or other implements you typically find in a gym, such as machines, dumbbells, barbells, and so forth.

The reason you want to load is because a big contributing factor to staying healthy and strong is having a good amount of muscle mass (don't mistaken this with being bulky), which enables you to be strong enough to move around, run, jump, squat, carry, push, pull, and pick things up off the ground. There seems to be a pattern that as we age, we tend to do what we know as cardio, which usually comes in the form of running. I think running is great, but for a holistic package we should be moving some sort of load often to increase, sustain, or at the very least slow down atrophy (muscle loss) as we age.

The way I like to explain strength to people, when looking at it over a long haul, is this: Think about the effort it takes you to walk up a flight of stairs today. It's usually surprisingly exhausting, no matter who you are. But, think about it. Who do you think is going to have an easier time climbing the stairs? Who do you think doesn't feel as fatigued or achy after? The person who has been lifting weights and doing some style of conditioning? The person who only runs? Or the person who doesn't do anything? Well, let's talk about it.

Imagine all three people are identical triplets. The strength and conditioning triplet is Alpha, the running-only triplet is Beta, and the person who doesn't do any physical activity is Omega. They are all 5 foot10, 170 pounds, with the same limb proportions, muscle build up etc. Alpha, who is squatting, deadlifting, and doing some sort of conditioning, is increasing both his strength and aerobic capacity. Your aerobic capacity is your ability to sustain workloads that typically require you to breathe heavier. While

Alpha is increasing his strength, his whole body gets stronger, so taking one step becomes less of a strenuous task on the body.

Now, imagine Beta, who only does cardio. He is building up some aerobic capacity, but if running is all he does, then his body will adapt to that particular stimulus. Stairs will still be relatively easy, but if he is not as strong as Alpha, then each step will be slightly more strenuous on the body. Even though they weigh the same, Alpha has much stronger and enduring legs, so moving his body up a set of stairs is less stress on his body versus Beta's. Now Omega, because he hasn't done any form of training, will find stairs the hardest. His heart rate and breathing rate will spike much higher than the other two because his body isn't used to dealing with any physical stress at all.

Climb for fitness

This actually reminds me of a quick story. Sam and I were walking with someone—let's call him Delta—at beautiful High Park in downtown Toronto. There's a big dog park with closed-off trail where you can let your dog off leash. It's really nice in the summer as you see all the big trees around you. At the bottom of the trail is a small stream that some dogs love jumping into, even though it smells sour at some points. The whole trail is about a 1.6km long and it loops around a big part of the park that is currently fenced off to try and let nature be, well, nature.

Delta and I were having a great conversation. About halfway through the trail, there is an uphill climb. I noticed Delta was becoming less responsive during our conversation. At first, I thought it was because I was talking too much, because I do that, but then when I looked over, I realized Delta was actually working really hard. He was trying to focus on his breath because of the hill we had just climbed. What was a casual walk for Sam and myself was a strenuous effort for Delta, which is great! I mean, I don't think Delta thought it was that great, but I can tell you right now that he started to walk a little more after that experience because he probably realized how important and effective walking can be as a means to getting in some fitness.

Now, Sam and I strength train often and we get out of breath a lot… on purpose. Crazy, right? Delta had never worked out a day in his life before that moment, and I would say he probably was not expecting what we said was going to be a fun leisurely walk to be a challenging task.

The next time you go for a walk, I suggest looking for a place that has some hills. When you walk up a hill, you are asking your body to work a bit harder. You work the glutes, hamstrings, and calves much more than you would on a flat road or trail. Not only does this make your muscles work harder, it is also great for increasing your cardio and gives your body a different challenge overall.

When walking on flat surfaces, you don't need as much strength. When climbing a hill, even if it is a small one, stronger people are going to have an easier time with it and not be as winded once they get to the top. Even though we might associate heavy breathing with cardio, I can tell you right now, strength training can do the same. It just depends on how you do it. Mixing both elements for me is something I'm a bit more biased towards as I think it has more transfer into everyday living (remember taking out the trash?).

The reason I am a fan of mixing both strength and conditioning is because there are benefits that I think serve people well both physically and mentally. For one, it could to not only increase muscular strength and muscular endurance but overall cardiorespiratory capacity, which has its own set of benefits. It also just allows people to have some variation in their program so they don't feel like they are doing the same thing over and over again. The realities are that we never have any clue what life is going to throw at us or which challenges we would like to take on, so we might as well become as strong as possible.

READER EXERCISE 11: Vice Grip

A lot of us are very familiar with conventional strength training where people do bicep curls or bench press. I challenge you to try something different, like a loaded carry! You can grab a pair of dumbbells, or maybe load some bricks into two backpacks and carry it for sixty seconds. If it was subjectively easy, try more weight and go again for another sixty seconds! Such a simple exercise but is has incredible benefits.

Post it on Instagram and use the hashtag #trainingforlife.

BUILDING A HEDGE

What is your hedge?

OR THE SAKE OF this chapter, your "hedge" is essentially an investment in yourself that will buffer you from any potential loss in future health and fitness. CrossFit® does a great job of explaining this in its "What is Fitness?" article, which is free to read online. The writer talks about a sickness–wellness–fitness continuum. Essentially, the fitter and healthier you get, the further you push yourself away from becoming decrepit or sick. If you have high levels of health and fitness, if something were to happen to you, instead of going from a state of wellness and getting closer to sickness, you are going from a state of fitness closer to a state of wellness. Of course, this is contextual for each individual but, as I have been training folks for more than a decade, I can see how true this continuum is.

From time to time, I have come across people who sincerely don't care to exercise, to look or feel a certain way, and really don't have any goals. For some of you, that might sound crazy. To others, it makes sense. I wonder if it's because the ideologies that come with the fitness world such as, "no pain, no gain," "you have to make sacrifices to get results"... Even just those two phrases can push people away. I think it's important to mention that anyone who steps into the fitness space knows, that those extremes are not necessary. By "fitness space," I am referring to something you are doing to improve your physical or mental health that involves moving your body for the sake of bettering yourself. This includes is strength, flexibility, endurance, sport, or anything for that matter. It can be done at home too, like a movement snack consisting of two minutes of burpees, or at the gym if it calls for a 90-minute session.

I think what isn't talked about enough is "building a hedge" against things that you might not be able to control, such as accidents. Maybe you were born with an autoimmune disease, or an unexpected health condition occurs. But what is within our control is an opportunity to reduce our chances of getting sick and slowing down decrepitude. You don't need to work out to fit someone else's ideals, just your own. The issue is that what we often see, is people are pushing for the "get your six pack abs now" and "this is how you will find happiness and elite health." This creates so many issues in the fitness world, which often lead to many mental health issues. What I propose is that if you don't have any goals, at least do something for the sake of the what ifs.

What can a fitness hedge do for you?

At my gym, we had an amazing person named Eddie join us as a member. Eddie came in with such crazy work ethic, which resulted in him being really fit. He could run, jump, do lots of reps of bodyweight movements, and was starting to get strong with the weights. After a short while, I also learned that he was a top Muay Thai fighter at one point. Muay Thai is a sport where two people get into a boxing-type ring and go head to head in a fight. Unlike traditional boxing where you can only use your fists, Muay Thai fighters use pretty much all of their limbs. They can hit you with their fists, elbows, shins, and one you don't want landed on you—a good knee. These athletes are extremely well-conditioned.

To sum it up, he was really fit. One day during class, we were going over technique for one of the Olympic lifts. After the class, Eddie said his lower back was bugging him. As a trainer, I put lots of care into making sure someone progresses well to avoid injuries. I remember talking with him at a BBQ we had later and he was holding his back. Something obviously was hurting beyond what seemed normal. It got to the point where he needed to go to the hospital because his legs started to go numb.

After all the examinations, the doctors told him that he had a tumor growing on his mid spine. There was really only one option: to have it surgically removed. That meant Eddie's chances of walking again were slim to none. This is extremely hard to accept for someone who has been so active his entire life. I personally still can't fathom it. After the procedure, the doctors told Eddie's wife he had zero chance of ever walking again... they told Eddie he had maybe a five per cent to give him a bit of hope. After the procedure, Eddie had to use a wheelchair to get around, which was a complete change from what had been used to.

Now, whether you are currently an athlete or someone who is able to freely stand up from your chair to the washroom, imagine having that taken away from you. This will do more than just affect your body, but also your mind. After a couple of years, I was fortunate enough to start working with Eddie and getting him back in the gym so he could start strength training and get some fitness in! Eddie's wife actually dropped into the gym for a class and I asked her how he was. She mentioned he was just struggling to find a way to work out. I accepted the challenge.

When Eddie came in for his first session with me, I was actually quite surprised as I knew he was initially in a wheelchair. He came in walking with ski poles! I was super-pumped to see that. Naturally, it created some curiosity as to how he was able to start to stand up right and use some support to get him from point A to point B.

When you are a personal trainer for someone for years, you have lots of solid conversations, and some people can truly become good friends which also allowed me to go more in depth with his injury. One day, Eddie and I were talking about his rehabilitation process and how that looked for people with spinal-cord injuries. One thing he mentioned was how many doctors told him how fortunate he was to be in such good shape before the procedure as it allowed him to start rehabbing right away. Eddie told me that a lot of people who didn't exercise before something life-changing like a spinal cord injury could have a much harder time at rehab. A fair number of people who were either obese or didn't have the muscle mass to support their body could not do some of the exercises required to make you get better quicker. A good example, would be trying to use parallel bars for physiotherapy. Parallel bars are a piece of equipment that act as railings on either side of your body. When a lot of patients are learning to walk again, they support their upper body on these railings and try to move their legs, whether there is some assistance or not. Supporting your body weight for most people is not an easy feat, hence why many have to do some extra work before starting the process. Eddie built himself an opportunity to start the rehab process a little bit faster than most people who are in similar situations.

You see, Eddie had been building his hedge for so many years. He was living an active lifestyle that paid dividends for his personal situation. Even though it is an unfortunate circumstance, his fitness is what bought him many years of life and put him years ahead of the rehabilitation process.

When I reached out to Eddie, I didn't have any intention of doing any work to strengthen his legs. But when I did a little test with something called the seven-way hips, I saw some potential to at least add a little bit of strength work. One of my personal favourite moments was when I saw Eddie contract his hamstring (back of the thigh) on his own. I became really excited as I saw this as a breakthrough. Basically, we had created an incline bench, where one side of the bench would be propped up onto a twenty-inch box. Eddie would then go on it upside down, so his feet were above his hips. If you have ever seen a hamstring curl machine at a gym, we tried to create something similar, but because there wasn't any strength in his hamstring, we used gravity. So, I would gently guide Eddie's foot towards his bum while he tried to do it on his own. After weeks of this exercise, there was one repetition where the muscle actually hardened and turned on—what we call a contraction.

Naturally, when a coach reaches a certain point with a client, we want the client to progress. When I saw Eddie contract his hamstring, we started to play around a little bit more to see what other exercises he could do. We progressed him to doing deadlifts, a movement where you pick up a barbell from a spot below your hips and stand up with it until you are fully upright with the bar. Another breakthrough! Eddie started to feel his hips and hamstrings, and I recall around that time he felt stronger.

Eddie would show me videos of himself walking up a hill with his ski poles and told me that he was feeling much stronger when he would walk. I would argue that even though Eddie couldn't kick your head anymore, he is much stronger and fitter today than he was the day after his surgery simply because of how much fitness and health he had to rely on.

Some days are easier than others. However, you start to learn that fitness, like the stock market, has highs and lows. But if there's one thing we know, it's that there is usually a positive return in the market over a long haul. If you stay patient and keep investing for the long term, a low in five years from now is what a high might be for you tomorrow. The goal is to have a nice steady climb, keep investing in your health, and build that hedge as wide and as tall as you can make it.

I genuinely want everyone in this world to do the things that bring them joy for as long as possible. Whether this is hiking through trails, fishing with your friends or quite simply, taking out your own garbage. If you get tired after a thirty-minute hike right now, in your current state, then a thirty-minute hike will be much more difficult for you in twenty to thirty years. If your back hurts after you catch a big fish now, then it will hurt much more in twenty to thirty years. But if you start to make some deposits on a consistent basis, starting today—then you will be very surprised at what you are capable of when those moments come at some point in the future.

READER EXERCISE 12: Hedge Plan

Write a list of five potential things that might require you to be fit. It could be saving someone's life, recovering from a disease or injury, or anything of that nature. Don't just think what can happen tomorrow but what can happen in ten, twenty, and even forty years from now.

Post your list to Instagram and use the hashtag #trainingforlife.

RANGE OF MOTION

CAN YOU TOUCH YOUR toes from a standing position? Can you reach over your head with straight arms without pain? If the answer is yes to both, you might be doing better than most people who neglect taking care of their bodies. Decrepitude is ultimately what we are trying to avoid with everything I am talking about in this book. Decrepitude is essentially the state of becoming older and losing function, being worn out due to age and neglect. Having a full range of motion among joints is super important for independence and health. I mentioned that strength training is important in order to work through a full range of motion with weights, but it is equally important to increase range of motion in general throughout your joints to enhance day-to-day living.

Why would you want to do this in the first place? It allows your muscles to stay healthy, improve blood flow, and feel less stiff. It also can be quite relaxing to your muscles, which can reduce overall stress. This may help create resiliency when you do ask for various activities from your body—most of which are often day-to-day tasks. Admittedly, the science is relatively light on stretching, but still quite promising on the benefits to the human body.

Human proportions

Before I dive too deep into it, it's important to understand that all of our bodies are built differently. Some of us have shorter torsos and long limbs or vice versa. Others have long arms and shorter legs or vice versa. This can all affect how you use your body to its full potential. What dictates whether or not we have longer limbs, torsos, and whatnot is based on an old painting named *The Vitruvian Man*, which was created by an old Italian artist from the 1400s named Leonardo da Vinci. Da Vinci painted this as a reflection of what he thought were ideal human proportions. *The Vitruvian Man* is now seen in many shapes and forms and it is still taught today in anatomy courses as a golden ratio of human proportion.

The reason I talk about proportions is because what might be a safe range of motion for me, might not be a safe range of motion for you. Yet, I believe everyone should learn how to increase their mobility and flexibility in a safe and effective way. Why is it vital? Well, in order to do everyday tasks on our own, we need to have the ability to move through some pretty big ranges of motion. Let's use grocery shopping as an example. If you can't safely reach down to the bottom shelf because of stiffness, you are losing your ability for maximum independence. You need the ability to change levels and grab the things you need for your everyday life.

Have you ever heard of someone who pulled her back while picking up something off the floor like a set of keys? It happens because of weakness but also because it's probably not a range of motion she is used to. We can use safe setting to improve the function of that range. Now, I am aware that the conventional way to picking up a set of keys might not be the same as the way you actually work out, but you should have the ability to move your body through that range of motion.

Good body parts to focus on

There are two areas that I would emphasize when it comes to increasing range of motion: the shoulder region and the hip region. Shoulder and hip joints are called "ball and socket" joints. If you were to look at your skeleton, you would see that your upper arm has a circular end that goes into your shoulder socket, which kind of holds it together like a suction cup.

Your hip is very similar in regard to how it is set up, except the upper thigh is the part that has that circular shape and your hip acts as the suction cup.

There seems to be one common culprit hidden right before our eyes that has been damaging our bodies for many years now: sitting. We tend to work for seven to ten hours a day, depending on our lifestyle. It makes our hips and hamstrings feel tighter, which can cause restrictions in those areas. Sitting can pull our shoulders forward, and when you try to use your body fully, you discover that things just don't feel right. All this sitting is what's crushing your body. Sitting in itself isn't the worst thing in the world, but when you are stuck in one position for roughly thirty-five-plus hours a week, your body is going to adapt to make it easier for it to remain in that position.

I find the first thing I need to do with people when they come into the gym is teach positions that are often the opposite of what most people are doing on a day-to-day basis. What's the opposite of sitting? A lot of movements that require us to have our shoulders back, our hips fully opened. All in all, just move into positions that you might not be used to. When you start to use your body in a different way, it gets a wake-up call. That's why it's always best to start off slow, light, and controlled.

I don't think you need to wait until you get into the gym to unglue your body from long-term positions. There are strategies you can implement into your everyday life to ensure you are keeping the body feeling nice and loose without always having to rely on a trainer. In fact, it is quite simple: get into the opposite position of what you are currently doing. So, if you are sitting down, try changing positions every twenty or so minutes. You can simply stand up, reach your arms over your head, and slightly overextend the belly to open it up. Do something as simple as that for one to two sets of twenty to thirty seconds, and it will start to make a difference. If you truly do that every twenty minutes, at the end of an eight-hour workday you would have stretched anywhere from eight to twelve minutes. Got to love movement snacks and how they add up.

This is an example of something most people can do. There are probably many other positions we are stuck in for long hours. Sitting seems to be the most common one. A reminder that no matter what position you are in, just do the opposite position a few times a day.

So how do you know if you are improving your range? Use a simple set of tests like I asked at the beginning of the chapter. Can you touch your toes? Can you reach overhead with straight arms without pain? Another simple hip test you can do is a squat test. Can you sit in a low squat position comfortably, with your hips below the knees, knees in line with the toes, and chest high for a couple of seconds or a couple of minutes? If you can, this shows sound function throughout the whole lower body, again, specifically in those hips. A good test for the shoulders is something called a wall angel. Place your back up against a wall and do a snow angel. Start with your arms at your sides and slide them up outwards along the wall until your upper arms are by your ears. Can you do this without arching your spine or taking your wrists off the wall?

These are a couple of very simple exercises you can do to see if your hips and shoulders feel good, but they also can help correct and strengthen them at the same time, which is pretty cool. Full range of motion is something we should strive to hold on to for as long as we possibly can to maintain independence. It will help you do simple daily tasks that you probably don't think about right now. Add in a little bit more movement at your workplace, especially if it is sedentary, and you will start to see some differences in how your body feels by the end of the day, week, and month.

READER EXERCISE 13: Stretch Break

Take a moment and think about which positions you hold most throughout your day. Set a timer ranging from twenty to thirty minutes. When the timer goes off, get into a position that looks like the opposite of what you are doing for thirty to sixty seconds.

Show us your stretch break on Instagram! Use the hashtag #trainingforlife.

HEALTH MARKERS

T HIS IS A FUN chapter to dig into. Mainly because at some point I need to contradict myself a little bit. Hopefully, you will get the overall message on using health markers to dictate how your body is functioning and if we need to stress about them at all. Health markers are the measurements of different systems that are working within your body, such as heart rate, blood pressure, and many others. I will stick to heart rate and blood pressure because those are a common one among folks.

When you visited the doctor in the past chances are that the doctor has taken your heart rate and blood pressure before. He is looking for normal values for you. In the health space, a heart rate between sixty to one hundred beats per minute (bpm) and blood pressure of 120/80 mmHg (mmHg is millimetres of mercury and is simply a unit of pressure) are considered "normal."

Build a strong heart
Let us start with the heart rate. Some doctors believe that fifty to seventy bpm is more of an ideal range, which I agree with to the fullest. I under-stand there might be some anomalies in the crowd. But just from personal experience, for someone who is trying to live a healthy long life, fifty to seventy bpm is a much safer range to be in because it is the sign of a strong heart, one that isn't working too hard to keep the body functioning.

The Women's Health Initiative did a major study that showed a twenty-six per cent increase in heart attacks and death in those with a resting heart rate of seventy-six bpm or higher compared to those with a lower resting heart rate. A slower heart rate can mean a couple of things. It can be an indication of your physical fitness, cardiovascular health, and just having a strong heart in general. There are always times where having a heart rate well below normal can also be an indication that something is wrong, such as heart disease or a heart infection.

My partner Sam is a competitive athlete; she does all the right things to improve herself. She eats well, sleeps well, and manages stress on a regular basis. When you measure her heart rate, it is a strong one (it's pretty low compared to "normal"). In high-school gym class, she tore a ligament in her shoulder called a labrum. She never thought to get surgery on it, but as she was getting stronger and stronger in college, her shoulder couldn't keep up with the loads. She made the tough decision to get it fixed.

I went with her to the hospital to support her and do whatever I could do to make her comfortable. The nurse was taking her pulse pre-surgery, which made me laugh quite a bit. The nurse mumbled to herself, "This can't be right" and redid the test. She was shocked and looked concerned for Sam's health. At first, I was concerned too, but when I noticed the nurse was checking the heart rate, I giggled a bit. Sam explained that she was a physically active person and that the heart rate the nurse was observing was a normal reading for her.

Now, we have to understand too that most nurses see people who are typically sedentary, which usually results in a higher heart rate. So anything that doesn't look closer to eighty to one hundred might actually be alarming, since, sometimes being below normal can be an indication that there can be complications.

That is one of the reasons I am very passionate about this book: the fact that it is normal to not have a resting heart rate be in what some experts consider an ideal range of fifty to seventy bpm is worrisome for me. It means there are too many of us who aren't taking care of the one thing we have for life, which is our bodies.

Another day, I was with a group of friends walking through a drugstore, and we walked by those machines where you stick your arm to get your heart rate and blood pressure measured. Personally, I've always loved those machines, probably because when I was young my grandmother would always measure herself and then make me do it. One of my closest friends sat down and got measured. When the results printed, I was worried, and I let him know. His resting heart rate was over one hundred bpm and his blood pressure was much higher than normal. I don't remember the exact figures, but it was enough for me to look at him and say, "Dude, some things got to change."

Thankfully, it was enough to motivate him to take action and put in some work to try and better himself. In a matter of months of hard work and having a new dog to walk, his numbers came down to what we would consider ideal. As a coach, I could see it through his energy levels. Even during his workouts, I could tell he was able to hold on to longer bouts of cardio and his strength was better. It was cool to see a correlation between some health markers and performance. I mentioned the dog because if you are walking your dog regularly you are actually doing yourself a huge blessing, which is simply walking for a good distance. You and your canine are reaping the benefits of exercise. As I mentioned earlier in the book, simply walking can have awesome benefits on what is happening inside your body.

There are many metrics we can use to determine if someone is getting healthier and adding years to their life. The reason I like heart rate and blood pressure metrics is because they are the easiest and most accessible to get. Nowadays you can download an app, take your heart rate instantly, and track it. If you don't want to download an app, you can find your pulse just by placing your index and middle finger together and putting them on the inside of your wrist below the thickest part of your palm. When counting resting heart rate, put on a fifteen- second timer, start with zero on the first count, and then count how many beats happen in that time frame. Multiply that number by four to get your resting heart rate.

There are some other health markers that are really important to keep track of; for most you likely have to go to the doctor and get blood work done to figure these out. Examples include things such as vitamin levels in your blood, triglycerides, and cholesterol. Vitamins are compounds found in food that allow your body so function at a better capacity. Triglycerides is a type of fat that gets stored in your fat cells when the calories you eat aren't used right away. Cholesterol tends to get a bad rap; it is also a fat-like substance but there is "good" and "bad" cholesterol and, in fact, we need cholesterol to help make hormones.

"But my uncle… and lived to 90"

There are so many factors to living a long life, it can almost be overwhelming. Now, this is the part of the chapter I might get some flak for and I am totally ready for it. It is time to contradict myself… a little. We have all heard those stories of someone's uncle who chewed cigarettes, slept for three hours a night, drank beer from morning to night, and lived to ninety. My question would be: "Did he have a *quality* life?" Oftentimes, people can do all the wrong things and live a long life, but then be under someone's care for twenty to thirty years because they didn't pay attention to their health.

Then you have the anomalies; people who go through physically and mentally damaging parts of their life which hurt them but they can still kick it without changing a single thing. In my life, that person is one of my grandfathers. I would put money down that my grandfather could drink anyone under the table; many have tried and many have failed. Ever since I was a kid, that man has always had a drinking problem, a "functioning" alcoholic, some would say. If you don't know him, you would think he is just a guy at a bar or a barbeque having a few. Really, those "few" are maybe his eighth or eleventh drink since he has been going at it all day.

I knew all this drinking would eventually catch up to him, and sometimes it did. My grandfather had some stomach issues, he puked a lot, but he never became decrepit. I don't wish poor on him, but you almost expect someone who takes such terrible care of themselves to eventually fall apart. He hasn't and it blows my mind. My mother and I had a scenario where he went into a bit of a panic attack, one that looked like a stroke, so we called the ambulance. At the hospital, we talked to the doctor and gave him the details of what had happened. Then the doctor gave us the rundown of the tests they would give my grandfather to see what was happening.

The doctor came to us and said something that until this day I can't believe. He looked at us and said, "Well, Jorge doesn't have any nutrients in his blood. He only has a bit of calcium." My grandfather would have one glass of milk every morning, so maybe that is what kept him going. Now, how crazy is that? He had survived on the calories from the beer for who knows how long. So, in a world where you have some people who do everything right to live to seventy without falling apart, you also have people who seem to do everything wrong. What is happening here?

After this little incident, my grandfather went back to my birthplace of Terceira, Acores. He didn't stop drinking, but he started to actually eat some real food, which brought him to a healthier weight according to the doctors in Portugal. The last time I went to Terceira and visited him, I was still impressed at his physical abilities. I think I know why he can still walk, carry things, laugh, and live alone without help. And from what I have seen from others who say their "uncles lived until one hundred chewing cigarettes," there are some similarities. The easy answer for me is genetics because genes do play a role with anything that has to do with the way our body is made up. However, when I look at the other parts of the picture, I think there are some factors that aren't necessarily noticeable.

I mentioned my grandfather can still walk, and when I say he walks, I mean he walks *everywhere*. He did it while he was here in Toronto, but he probably does it more now in Terceira. With all that walking, he also helps people out a lot, which usually results in him carrying relatively heavy items. And, yes, sometimes those are beer cases. On top of it, Terceira is a very hilly island. As you know from the story I told above, walking up and down hills, whether you are doing it with some sort of load or not, requires you to utilize more muscles. In my opinion, this is for sure preserving some quality muscle.

Another big factor to my grandfather's longevity (I'm sure) so far is that he has always managed to keep his weight down. It was really down when he wasn't eating, but even now with some food everyday he doesn't seem to be adding too much body fat. Keeping body fat in check has also been shown to increasing someone's lifespan. Now, add that with a stress-free island life, and I can understand a little bit more how someone can look like they are doing everything wrong, but still be thriving. Now, imagine how healthy he'd be if he had done everything right.

To conclude, we can use health markers to make change for the better to get us from a state of being sedentary and having higher-risk chances of disease, all the way to building a strong capacity in the heart and lungs and getting that body moving. Couple that with starting to eat well and managing stress and sleep and you have a pretty good recipe to living a longer happier life. Enjoy your time here and have a beer or two; just please move and eat some real food too.

READER EXERCISE 14: Health Check

Get your heart rate and blood pressure checked! Record it and then after a couple of months of exercising, take the measurements again and see if there are improvements!

Share with us on Instagram! Use the hashtag #trainingforlife.

GETTING OFF MEDICATION

MEDICATION HAS AN IMPORTANT role to play in the modern world, and it's why many people can still function as a part of society. Let's discuss specific medications people could get off of by changing their lifestyle choices, and how I would prefer them to do that instead, only using prescriptions or over the counter drugs as a short-term boost as needed.

When I say short-term, I don't necessarily mean two to four weeks; certain individuals need some prescriptions a little bit longer. One concern I have with our society is that instead of trying to fix the root cause of an issue with our bodies, that gets put on the back burner because there is some sort of pill that will push the symptoms aside as a temporary solution.

Let's begin with anti-inflammatory medications. Of course, they have a purpose. But if you have been dealing with back pain for two to three years and anti-inflammatories are your go-to, yet you haven't tried to fix the root cause, I believe there may be a better way to handle that. I am not a doctor, but I believe we need to look at what the root cause is and ask ourselves if there is a non-medication solution. The problem is, fixing the root cause requires effort. This is when we need to go back to the motivation–discipline–habit chapter and try to give ourselves a big "why" behind getting out of pain. Something really cool happens when these people come into the gym. They learn how to lift properly, how to engage their muscles effectively, and just get stronger overall to minimize the back pain and, better yet, even get rid of it!

Sometimes, it doesn't take a coach; it may be another health care professional in the therapy world that can help (I am sure if you ask around in your network you can find some solid professionals). The point is, if you are in pain for an extended period of time, it is worth checking out why, so it doesn't worsen over time. Some professions make this a little more difficult for sure. I think of my family and friends in trades like construction or mechanics, where they have to do awkward lifting on a regular basis that involve some weird twists and turns. For them, I usually suggest thoughtful and mindful lifting, although some of the lifting scenarios are not always ideal. People of all work places who require to lift objects, especially tradespeople should be trained better in how to move odd objects more effectively to avoid long-term pain, and maybe they cut down from six bottles of anti-inflammatories to one—hopefully zero.

Fitness can get you off medication!

This story about prescriptions is short but packs a small punch in it. I had a client who pulled me aside after I finished training a group and she seemed happy and excited to share some news. Not long before, she had a condition resulting in her having higher blood pressure than the normal range. The doctor prescribed some blood-pressure medication and told her she would have to use these pills, probably for the rest of her life. She mentioned that some of her family members also took the same prescription, which meant there as a high likelihood that the condition was genetic. She also said that all her life she had always tried different ways to stay in shape, such as riding her bike all the time, running, and so on. It wasn't until she started doing high-intensity circuit training (CrossFit® to be exact) that something started to change. She went for a check-up and the doctor had told her that she stop taking the medication.

How awesome is that? You are told you need to take medication forever and then you play around with different streams of exercise and find something that gets you off medication. Now, I'll be the first to say I am sure there are a number of lifestyle factors that could have also played a role, but the idea that if there is a chance to manage your body through lifestyle choices versus a prescription, the former is something I will always recommend. There has been a good amount of research to back up that under good supervision, high-intensity circuit training is quite effective to give someone a great dose of fitness but also improve health markers like blood pressure and lowering resting heart rate when compared to low-intensity circuit training.

Another really cool story comes from Sam. When Sam was younger, she was already quite active. She played many sports such as volleyball, soccer, and did racquet sports. Since she lived about an hour north of Toronto, which has much more greenery and forests, she did things like hiking and biking. The problem though, was she always felt like she had joint pain. She told me once she always thought she was hurt from the sports she was playing. If her hands or wrist started to bug her, she would throw on a wrist brace. If her knee was achy, then a knee wrap went around it. She even mentioned her gym teachers sometimes thought she was lying to get out of class, which was untrue.

When Sam checked out her aches at the doctors, she discovered she had juvenile rheumatoid arthritis, an autoimmune disease that causes inflammation within the joints, usually in those up to sixteen to eighteen years old. Sometimes the symptoms can disappear with treatment and some kids grow out of it. Any kid who gets juvenile rheumatoid arthritis might experience it for a different timeline, some maybe six weeks and others a lifetime.

When I met Sam, she was nineteen years old and still had symptoms of arthritis. When her hands were inflamed, you couldn't see her knuckles when she made a fist. To help keep inflammation down, she took a very strong dose of naproxen (anti-inflammatories), coupled with Losec, which is a medication used to treat gastroesophageal reflux disease. She took these medications for six years. The doctors did warn her that what she was taking was bad for her stomach lining. This didn't really sit well with Sam. When I met Sam, she did a fair amount of cardio and lighter-weight, high-rep work as she had aspirations of doing a physique show, which is a competition that exhibits muscular tone, build, and symmetry. After a little while, I started to help her with her barbell squat and taught her the

Olympic lifts at the gym of the school we met at. She started to take off with it and lift heavier weights and she began to do CrossFit as well.

When you want to get better at something sometimes, you're willing to make bigger jumps. I don't mean you start training three to four hours a day, but you start to eat better, your sleep habits improve, and you become more conscious of how you are moving, which is what Sam did. She started to get really strong and also weeded out foods that didn't really sit well with her. She started to notice that her inflammation wasn't as bad and made it a goal to get off the medication. Until this day, I remember going to a check-up with Sam; it was cool to sit beside her and hear the doctor say that the signs of arthritis were minimal, and that all her joints and bones looked stable. She is now off that medication.

I do want to note that getting off medication won't work in every scenario. We still need to trust recommendations made for us by professionals. My grandmother, who I mentioned in the beginning of the book, for example, had suffered from a subdural hematoma and needs to be on blood thinners for the rest of her life so she doesn't get another clog in her brain. I have friends with Type 1 diabetes who cannot survive unless they take insulin. These scenarios vary for every person and his or her unique experiences in life. But there are lifestyle choices you can make to potentially get off medications you don't need, nor do you like taking. It does require a couple of common things that we are stressing in this book: start finding a way to move your body.

READER EXERCISE 15: Restoration Plan

We all have things we do in the short-term to fix long-term pain. My challenge to you is find out what you do in the short-term that could be fixed by addressing the issue with exercise. Write a list of three things and start addressing them.

Post your list to Instagram and use the hashtag #trainingforlife.

HOW MUCH SHOULD I TRAIN?

I F YOU RECALL THE movement snack chapter, I talked about how we need seventy-five minutes of relatively more intense exercise and 150 minutes of moderate exercise per week. If you can break that up into chunks that work best for you, then do it. It is probably the best way to start and helps people ease their way into their own personalize fitness routine that fits their lifestyle. How much each individual should train is up to their personal goals and what they are trying to achieve. When it comes to training for life, I want you to find a system that works best for you. This may mean three days a week of one hour at the gym, followed by one day playing a sport. This can be four days a week of 45-minutes at the gym and then one day hiking. There is no cookie-cutter approach to exactly how you should do this.

I have observed people who have figured it out and others who are still in the pursuit of finding what works best. It starts with the quote I once saw on an Instagram post: "If you leave the gym feeling like you could have done more, that's a good sign." Some of you might have read that and thought, "But we have to go hard every day!"

No. No, you don't. In fact, if you are training for the sake of maintaining health and longevity then you never really need to reach certain thresholds, whether that be mentally or physically. You should only reach those thresholds if you wish. A good example I can give is I got invited by a friend of mine to try Brazilian Jiu Jitsu, which is a martial art based on ground fighting and submission holds. I am a fairly fit and competitive individual and I did quite well – to the point where one of the instructors mentioned if trained more I can be ready for a tournament. As someone who loves to compete, in that moment I thought, "I really don't want to." I just wanted to enjoy the sport as a means to get in shape versus pushing my limits on it. Who knows, maybe that will change one day. Point being, you don't need to reach the pinnacle of what you are doing to reap the benefits.

Lots of people may think that I don't want anyone pushing themselves whether that be in a sport they play or lifting weights by finding one to five rep maxes on exercises like deadlifts or presses or testing your baseline times that act as a benchmark to try and beat after a cycle of training (a good example is a 2,000-metre row).

I want to clarify that is not what I mean. If I am training a seventy-four -year-old woman or a young college student looking for function, I don't believe finding a one rep max serves them much. Yes, there are some master powerlifters who are extremely inspiring, and college athletes who want to go pro, but that's just not the norm. Most seventy-four-year-old women need a program they feel safe in. Most people in fact, like you and me need a method that allows us to feel more energized in our day to day living so we can be better partners, friends, parents and just be nicer to our bodies for the long haul – and more often than not, the answer comes back to just move often.

Now, the last thing I like doing is treating people like they are fragile. I have trained many people, young and old, who are quite impressive, but I have always had more success when I allow clients to stay within their psychological tolerances. In the strength chapter I talked about that client who was slightly older and was eager to lift that 185-pound yoke. Had she said, "I don't really feel comfortable lifting that today" as opposed to just trying like she did, then I would be prepared to have something else for her.

As a trainer, you want people to be in a safe space where they can get in some good fitness over the long haul, not just for today. Back to ". . . you could have done more, that's a good sign"—I love that because it keeps people hungry. Too often, I have come across people who crush themselves just because that's what they believe makes up a great workout and they do it way too often. Not to say pushing the limit is bad, but some people do it too fast, too often, and usually with no real direction, which can lead to injuries that are demotivating, if not restricting you from things you genuinely enjoy.

So, what is the best way to start? Movement snacks for one. If you haven't started training, go back and re-read that chapter and then start slow. Next, progress your environment, whether you plan on working out from home, a gym, with your sports team, outdoors, or a group fitness gym. There are so many different styles of fitness and the cool part about training for longevity is you can vary all of them. I challenge people all the time to try different things, safely, of course. No matter how or where you start, you need to take into account three things for any fitness program. Don't look at these three points as black or white: each one sits on a spectrum.

First is safety. For longevity, this is hands down the most important one for anyone who is looking to train for life. Now, let's really exaggerate what is safe and what is not. Assuming you have never done anything, we are going to look at sitting on the couch watching TV as very safe but extremely ineffective in getting you results that would push the needle forward in your fitness and health. On the opposite end, again assuming you have never done anything, you walk into a gym and you or a coach decides to do a series of exercises, pushing maximal weights, maximal intensity, and with zero instructions.

This would be a recipe for disaster. Instead, what we want for longevity is somewhere you can learn to move effectively and safely but still have a good plan to progress. An example of progressing at home might be adding a few more reps to your workouts because you need an extra challenge, or adding five minutes to your total workout time. The good thing about having a coach is that he can safely help you progress slowly over time if you communicate your goals effectively.

Next is efficacy, which simply means: Is what you are doing working? I like variance in my training, which I truly recommend for people who simply want to just have fun and train for life. Having something to test every once in a while is a fun way to measure your progress in variety of domains. It doesn't have to be crazy; it can be the tests from the longevity chapter, such as hanging off a pull-up bar for as long as you can or seeing how far you can perform a standing long jump. These small and simple tests can give you an idea if what you are doing is working.

It is important to realize that those who started training at a very young age eventually hit a point where some of our benchmarks won't be attainable. Or hitting them would actually put us out of commission for a little while. We will all reach a point where we don't necessarily get "fitter"; we are just trying to preserve as much as possible. After preservation mode, we begin to slow the aging process down as much as possible and try to hold onto all the muscle, range of motion, and abilities we have acquired. The cool thing is if you start TODAY, and you are at fifty per cent of that when you are eighty then even though you are slowing the process down you will still be much more well off than most. If you can run up a set of stairs in thirty in sixty seconds, and at eighty you can run up those stairs in 120 seconds, it is still way better than not getting up those stairs at all.

Lastly, how efficient is what you are doing in moving toward your goals? My favourite part of not having immediate goals is you can simply imply patience on your results because training for life is a very distant goal. If someone told me they want to add fifty to eighty pounds to one of their barbell lifts (this happens) in three to four months then I need to provide something that is very efficient, has high efficacy. But guess what usually suffers? Safety. When training for longevity we can dial back that goal to create something more distant, which might bring the efficiency and efficacy down to drive up the safety of the program. Maybe fifty to eighty pounds in two or three years would be a better-suited goal in some cases, and this depends on what the movement is, training background, etc.

Out of the three points I just mentioned, I would emphasize safety when it comes to deciding how much to do. You can train safely five to six days a week and see results, and you can train safely three to four days a week and see results. The important part about the frequency in which you decide to do something that looks and feels like exercise is consistency over a long haul. Don't stress about missing a day or two of being physical in a setting like a gym. Instead, build important habits like taking the stairs instead of the elevator so that even on days when you don't lift a physical weight you are still doing something that keeps your body moving.

When I first started training, I came into it with a competitive mindset, trying to get results very quickly and forcing numbers to get faster and higher. After a couple of years, what resulted was the beginning of dealing with nagging injuries that started to create setbacks. After a little while, you realize that you love to train for more than just results. Training really helps me mentally. I learned to focus more and more on quality as the years went by. I realized when your body feels great, that quality drives progress. What you get in return is more strength, better fitness, and optimal health.

It truly comes down to learning more about your body and how to listen to it. A reporter once asked a masters athlete (usually athletes over thirty-five) whose name slips my mind, how he was able to compete for such a long period of time. He said, "Don't wait until you're actually hurt before modifying workouts; listen for the little whispers and adjust accordingly."

So… How much should I train?

Regardless of what you do, start slow and gradually build up if find it adds to your life. If you join a group fitness program, start with two times a week for one to two weeks and then build up until you find something you can sustain. From experience this is usually three times a week.

If you go off on your own, here are recommendations to follow. Strength train two-three times per week. Do cardiovascular work two or more times per week. Stretch ten minutes a day.

For strength, keep the exercises basic. Squats, deadlifts, presses, and single arm rows to name a few. Pairing non-competing exercises can be great to create efficient workouts. These are called supersets. Two to four sets of eight to twelve reps is a great starting spot. Rest sixty to ninety seconds between sets. Add some core at the end and you are good to go.

Example:
3 sets of:
12 Dumbbell Goblet Squats
8 Dumbbell bench press
-rest 90 seconds-

3 sets of:
12 Dumbbell Deadlifts
8 Dumbbell rows per arm
-rest 90 seconds-

3 sets of:

30 sec forearm plank

30 sec suitcase carry per arm (single arm farmers carry)

-rest 90 seconds-

For cardio, you can start with something that is low impact. I am a fan of a bike to start. Twenty minutes at a continuous pace.

The above are examples of what you can do to begin. Regardless of how you start, you would slowly build up in load and/or volume over time to progress.

READER EXERCISE 16: Safety list

How much each of us trains is going to vary, but safety is super important if you are training for a long time. Write down a list of three things you will do to ensure you have a safe training journey.

Share your list on Instagram and use the hashtag #trainingforlife

INJURIES

I F YOU HAVE A fear exercising because of injuries, I can assure you that not exercising will leave you in far worse condition. You need to decide if you would prefer to potentially have aches from exercising, or aches from being sedentary. The difference is exercise mitigates the risks of metabolic disease while being sedentary will bring on a host of problems that are currently the leading causes of death in North America.

A lot of times when you ask people what is holding them back from starting a fitness routine there are a couple of common answers. The first one is not having enough time, but we now know how to fill small gaps in our day with a little bit of movement to sneak in some fitness no matter where we are. Another big reason is because people fear getting injured. It's a fair reason; no one wants to get hurt. Injuries can come in many shapes and forms, and there are ways to avoid them.

Acute and chronic injuries

Acute injuries are usually quick and sudden. When I used to play soccer, I got injured in a knee-on-knee collision. When I let my knee heal well, I never struggled with that injury again. That is an example of an acute injury.

Chronic injury, by comparison, is when muscles and ligaments do not heal well and can start to create some muscle imbalances, tightness, or even weakness at some locations of the body. These usually happen over time.

To give you another example from when I was playing soccer, I sprained my left ankle. Being stubborn, I never fully rehabilitated it and re-sprained it again and again. When I started to lift weights, I had lots of stiffness in that ankle and even when I got some range of motion back, I had to work really hard to make it strong again.

If you have ever played a sport or want to play sport, I have something to say that is not popular at all. It is not a matter of IF you get hurt, it's a matter of WHEN. The first time I said it's a matter of WHEN, I remember the couple of people around me were upset like I was being negative, yet every person in that room was dealing with an injury related to our sport. Too many of today's sports have elements that can bring forth an injury, and a lot of times it starts when we are just kids. Growing up playing soccer, I ended up losing count of the number of knee injuries I saw. If those athletes didn't rehab properly, they would probably be the ones telling me that "squats hurt my knees."

How to avoid injury

If you are training for life, and longevity is the goal, everything you do should prevent you from getting injured. That usually means staying within your limits both mentally and physically. Even if you are an athlete, what you do in the gym should be preventative work so you can become more resilient in your sport. The stronger you become, whether the weights you lift, or the new range of motion you reach, the endurance you train, you going to become more resilient or at least, speed up your recovery if you get hurt. For most of you reading this right now, life is your sport so you must become resilient to life. Remember, when you plan on doing something like fitness for a long time, you need to have an incredible amount of patience when it comes to progressions, so you can keep yourself as safe as possible.

Ego is often our biggest enemy when we step into the gym. Very rarely do I see people not struggle with their ego, and it's usually out of pure joy for what they are doing. We start to get excited with what our bodies are capable of and immediately want to keep testing and pushing the limits. Usually when we do this, we start to deviate from quality movement if we are pushing too hard. Now, I don't want you to take this as never push yourself because progressing over time is key. I once heard Pavel Tsatsouline give some solid insight. (Tsatsouline is a coach in the fitness industry who is most known for his introduction of the kettlebell in the late 1990s and since then has produced multiple books on minimalistic training.) In a podcast, Tsatsouline said that there was a time where the old school Soviet strength athletes would use the same weight on the barbell for weeks until it became subjectively easier. Once the barbell would feel lighter or the athletes could move faster after a while, they would add some weight. When you do this over time, it is called progressive overload, which is essentially a gradual increase of stress on the body.

A lot of Tsatsouline's training methods are extremely simple and tackle a lot of the elements that help people with longevity. And while we are on that topic, I do believe a kettlebell is one of the best tools you can start with if you decide to work out from home.

Solidifying your gains (using the same load for a few weeks) is a great way to avoid injuries. Another thing we should take into account is that it's okay to do different things to avoid overuse injuries. Take running for example. A lot of runners, mainly those who like to cover many kilometres in a week, tend to put lots of stress on their bodies. This can result in some sort of knee or hip pain. People who love running can benefit quite a bit from doing strength training to become more resilient. This might mean they need cut back on the kilometres to dedicate some time to getting stronger. Remember: strength training is that one thing that we should all be doing if we want to become more resilient.

Not long ago, I started to work with someone who wanted to compete in an Ironman Triathlon. She came to me with an incredible background. She had done ultra-marathons, which are essentially runs that go beyond 42 kilometres. She mentioned to me that she does a lot more trail running now because the concrete leaves her pretty banged up after a while, and she was dealing with some minor injuries here and there. When I took over all of her programming, I made some changes that definitely looked and felt very different for her. Now before I go on, someone training for an Ironman has very different short-term goals than someone who simply training for life. The ideas are the same, just on a different level.

When we started to work together, I immediately started having her strength train in addition to her Ironman disciplines: swimming, cycling, and running. After months of work, we started to test different distances and she was crushing it while setting personal records. The most important part for me, though, was that she said she felt so much more resilient. Things like running on concrete didn't beat her up like before. A big reason for this is because we started to strengthen muscles and tendons required for her to do her sport effectively without feeling broken. We also added sessions that involved more sprint efforts. These changes in someone's training can make a huge difference between surviving in their sport versus thriving.

This can be the same for those who just want to be healthy! Say you start to fall in love with running and you want to run five days a week. I challenge you to start running three times a week and spend the other two days focusing on strengthening your body. This will allow you to enjoy running for much longer in your life. These are general recommendations. Ultimately, you need to find what is going to work for you while always thinking about the most sustainable approach, which may not look the way you want.

The objective should always come back to quality over quantity to avoid giving yourself any type of injuries but understand that you cannot always escape them. Sometimes they come at times you aren't even expecting them such as picking up your kids, or a piece of paper on the floor. If you are getting started lifting weights, a good tip is to think of any injury you have had in the past and be nice to that area to begin. Ask yourself questions like if you have a job that requires you to do the same movement over and over again. Do you sit for long periods of time? Have you ever fallen? These can all contribute to potential future discomfort. Again, there are so many reasons why you could potentially get injured. The cure: Build your hedge.

At the end of the day, we must all do our own risk assessment and stay within certain boundaries if longevity is the goal. I love the idea of solidifying your gains, doing things with quality over quantity, and varying what you are doing if that means you get to do what you actually enjoy for much longer. Training smart and staying injury free is the goal.

READER EXERCISE 17: Solidify your body

There are methods and systems in place that might help you prevent injury. A simple one mentioned is solidifying your gains. For the next three weeks, to solidify your gains, do what you have been doing; don't change it. Follow the same reps and sets or volume, which should feel subjectively easier or lighter than the session before. Learn from it. After three weeks, add five to ten pounds. Do this often and the strength you will build over a long haul will surprise you.

Try this out and let us know how it goes and what you felt. Post on Instagram and use the hashtag #trainingforlife.

OBSTACLES & CONSISTENCY

WHEN WE TALK ABOUT obstacles, I am not thinking about things like the American Ninja Warrior race you might have seen on TV but things that people consider real-life obstacles. This ranges from topics like injuries, to time, work, kids, vacations, family duties, and so forth. A lot of these things are just part of everyday life, so we must learn to put strategies in place to prevent us from falling off what we are trying to do. We need to remember that we are one workout and one meal away from getting back on track. After coaching for many years, I sometimes come across people who are consistent in different parts of the year. That is usually when we see solid progress. Now, if you take a bit of time off the gym to go and do something different such as focus on a sport then that's awesome. But what can you do if you enter a period of time that you are not exercising at all?

Find accountability

I have this one gentleman in the gym who is like that. He's really fit, works hard in and outside of the gym, but is present in spurts. When I talk to him, there always seems to be something going on, whether it is work, or taking care of his newborn. There have been times where he will be gone from the gym for a month or two. But when he is back, it is like he never left. He is there full force and working hard every day. He knows he can workout at home and sometimes he probably does, but he loves working out with people. I have noticed this with a handful of people who struggle to exercise on their own. They just need a friend or a group of people they can work out with. A lot of times, the reason people in group class settings come back is because they have a friend or two that message them, "Hey, where are you? Let's workout." That short message helps keep people accountable and coming back. They are your accountability buddies.

If you struggle with taking initiative to do something, find a group of people to hold you accountable. It can be super powerful in helping you create consistency when it comes to finding ways to continue to move throughout your day. This is also another pro of working with a coach!

Build a home gym

A lot of times when life happens, it is usually something that is time-consuming. Naturally, the first thing to go is any travel to a gym. Which is why I believe everyone should start to acquire a home gym for themselves and their family. A lot of people think home gyms are ridiculously expensive but guess what? They are not. Looking back in the movement snack chapter, if you recall, I started working out at home with some pushups and sit-ups. Your body is your home gym. Find a spot where that you can deem your "movement" area and create a space where fitness or stretching is what goes down. A good place to find basic equipment to add to your home gym is your local dollar store, where you can find things like light dumbbells, foam rollers, and skipping ropes. It's actually quite impressive how much exercise equipment costs less than $10.

You can also ask friends and family if they have anything they don't use and start there. If you decide to put more money into your home gym, think about the things you would use the most. I usually recommend some weights first, starting with kettlebells because of their space efficiency. Some people prefer going with a bar and a set of weight plates. Over time, you can start to build quite an impressive home gym whether you live in a condo or a big house. Having this set in place reduces the excuses you can have. A home gym coupled with movement snacks enables you to get fitness in often. Instead of three to five minutes of squats and sit-ups, you can easily pick up a skipping rope and do three to five minutes of skipping mixed with something else. So not only does your home improve, but you have other fun options for movement snacks too.

Maybe you are that friend who holds a lot of people accountable and has a home gym. This can be really fun because you can have people come over, grab some equipment, and create a partner workout. Get after it for twenty minutes and then sit down to eat some brunch and enjoy some coffee.

Have a long-term goal

One of the last things I recommend for getting either through or over an obstacle to get back on track is to remember your long-term goals—or create one. Having a goal that is in the distant future is a very easy way to stay on track for the long term. We will build on this on the next chapter.

READER EXERCISE 18: Build your home gym

If you don't have any equipment at home, I challenge you to purchase one piece you can use often. It might be a skipping rope you can get for pretty cheap! Maybe ask a friend if they have any old kettlebells or dumbbells laying around. Next, rope in someone into a workout with you and try to hold each other accountable in case one of you falls off.

Post your piece of equipment to Instagram! Use the hashtag #trainingforlife.

GOALS

TO START, I AM really happy to get to the goals chapter. Why? Because it was my goal. Getting to this chapter signifies the effort in making this book a reality versus just an idea. For some, goal-setting is quite difficult. But maybe I take it for granted because I have made and reached many goals in my life so far. I have also come up short on others. I want to teach you a different way to look at goals, but before we get there, I think it would be irresponsible if I didn't start with a goal-setting technique that has worked for many people. And when you are exposed to the fitness industry, it gets drilled into your head.

Some of you might already be familiar with SMART goals: specific, measurable, attainable, realistic, time-oriented. It's an easy acronym to remember that has all the key components of what it takes to write down goals whether they are short term or long term.

1. Specific

The specific part of SMART goals is, in my opinion, one of the most important ones because it needs to be action- based. You can't just say, "I want to lose weight." You need to be much more detailed in how you are approaching this goal. To lose weight requires us to usually eat in a calorie deficit, which means we are consuming less calories than our bodies are burning that day. In order to do this, you probably need to keep track of your food for a short while and prepare meals. It is also beneficial to give yourself a number to chase so that when you achieve that goal you can reset. So, a good specific goal might sound like this: "I will lose ten pounds in three months by tracking my food and meal prepping every Sunday.

2. Measurable

You want something you can measure your progress with. To build on the example above, use a scale to measure your body weight to see if you are going in the right direction. When it comes to weight loss versus fat loss, there is something important to think of. For instance, if you are using exercise to help with fat loss, note that when moving weights you will build denser muscles, so it can appear that you aren't moving down much on the scale. One pound of muscle is physically denser than a pound of fat. Weight loss assumes you are just trying to cut down as much as possible, which of course accounts for body fat, but muscle mass and water weight could be lost as well. Even though what we are talking about is an example of SMART goals, I know there tends to be frustration with fat loss when it seems like you are doing everything to bring the number on the scale down.

3. Attainable

Attainable is something that is within your scope. If you want to lose thirty pounds in thirty days, that is something that is extremely difficult and likely not attainable. You may have heard of someone doing it, but I guarantee you it is rare, doesn't benefit long-term habits, and it is not good for you. In addition, if a big obstacle comes next week and now you have to order in and miss the gym for a couple of days, this can affect how attainable your goals are. It is recommended that one to two pounds is a safe amount to lose per week. So, a good thirty-day weight-loss goal is somewhere between four to eight pounds, depending on the individual and where she currently is at in terms of bodyweight.

4. Realistic

Realistic brings up the question: Is it actually possible to do what you wish in the time frame, given your personal circumstances? This one is just about being honest with yourself. Do you believe your goal is realistic—right now? Are you willing to do the work and create the habits necessary to make it a possibility?

5. Time-oriented

Lastly, the time in which you wish to complete this goal. If the end result is three months away, you should also create an action plan that helps you attain your goal. For example, you can use Sundays to make meals for the week, create a checklist of how many times you will hit the gym, or how much water you'll drink. Creating a weekly plan keeps you focused. Instead of just thinking about three months down the road, you can do things that matter right now. This will make your goals not feel so distant. Focusing on what you can do with your time in the short term is super beneficial because you can stay present and truly learn the process of what it takes to sustain your goals even after you have reached them.

This is the conventional way to learn how to goal set and I do believe it to be a super effective way to start creating and attacking these milestones. I also think how we choose our goals are important, not just for our physical health but for our mental health. Using the example of losing ten pounds in three months, I would ask someone why they chose this goal. If the answer is, "because I want six-pack abs," then two things come to mind. One: there is nothing wrong with that. Two: are you okay if you lose that six-pack? The reason I say this is because age is inevitable; it is the one thing no one can change. In this life, we will experience many different changes to our bodies. What may seem like an ideal physique, might not be sustainable when we are older. I find people who have aesthetic goals seem to be the hardest on themselves over the years when they start to get older.

I have nothing against aesthetic goals, but I do believe at some point we have to be okay with releasing from the pressures of looking a certain way and instead put more emphasis on active daily living. One of the best bodybuilders of all time, Dorian Yates, was interviewed on a podcast and he said something that everyone who trains for aesthetics should hear. When he retired from his bodybuilding career because he knew he couldn't sustain his size or physique, he was totally okay with getting back to a size and physique that would be healthier for him. He knew that in order to have longevity and health, he couldn't sustain the level of training that he was doing because it would affect his personal life later on. He embodies something that I think about a lot myself and have talked to some others about: Have the big picture in mind, even when chasing short-term goals.

When you have a goal, go for it. Given that I am talking about training for life, maybe most of you don't care about having six-pack abs or chasing a 300 to 400 pound squat, and that's fine. But those goals are often quite attainable when people pick very specific goals, and that's great. Implementing something like the SMART approach will help many get there. But a lot of times, whether it is a number on a barbell or competing at a high-level competition, what is needed to get achieve results is oftentimes not the most sustainable approach to longevity. Ultimately, a combination of both is great. Use the SMART goals to achieve those three-/six-/nine-month goals, but always keep in the back of your mind that at the end of the day, longevity is the key.

Another athlete who really sticks out to me is Cristiano Ronaldo, a Portuguese soccer player who has countless records and trophies, both as an individual and with a number of top European teams. When you are a soccer player, you live your life in seasons and tournaments, and you want to be as prepared as possible for each game and each season. Many players only play for about eight to ten years. Some stretch their careers out to twelve to fourteen years, but that is pretty rare. What is important to note is that the player's quality usually decreases the longer he plays.

There are some important factors to note as to why these players are not as good. It could be age, maybe they are not training as much, sleep quality can alter their performance, or perhaps they are more relaxed with their diet. Ronaldo has always said that he eats only good food, he trains safely and effectively, and puts a lot of emphasis on recovery. This has allowed him to play at the top level for more than eighteen years. It honestly doesn't look like he is going to stop anytime soon. The things Ronaldo did when he was younger is now paying dividends in his sport. He had short-term goals, but also always had his career longevity in the back of his mind.

I don't expect anyone to train like an athlete. But if you build all the good habits right now, you can build a big hedge against decrepitude and sickness, and then you can live a very happy and long life. Whether you are an athlete, a parent, or a child, you all have one goal in common that is distant in the horizon—your health—for some of us twenty, forty, maybe even sixty years away.

So, my question to you is this: What are your goals when you are eighty years old?

RECAP

LONGEVITY: On average, the human population is starting to live longer lives with the benefits of having better access to clean water, food, shelter, and a robust medical system. But we can do a better job as a society try to create a more quality life for ourselves. The answer to that usually comes from learning more about what we need to work on and what are the big bang-for-your-buck categories. Strengthening your core, not just the front but the sides and the back as well, is vital to having long-term strength.

Building a stronger grip over a lifetime is extremely beneficial when it comes to everyday living and having the ability to move items from point A to point B. Having strong legs ensures you can walk up and down stairs, sit and stand with ease, and have good balance. Developing those faster muscles fibres that help us react quickly, jump and sprint. This is good to keep muscle quality as high as possible as we age. Lastly, we need to take care of our brain. Exercise does this, but also just challenging yourself with different activities, eating good food, and managing stress.

FITNESS OUTSIDE OF THE GYM: Don't get sucked into the idea that the only way to get into shape or test yourself has to be in the gym. Ultimately, no one is going to care how much you can lift, or how fast you can run. Hiking, climbing mountains, going to different lakes or beaches in your area, and having the ability to play sports on the beach or with family, whether they are young or old, will always yield better memories. You also never know when fitness can save your life, and that usually doesn't happen in the four walls of a gym. Get out and enjoy the body you have.

MOVEMENT SNACKS: These small bouts of movement sprinkled throughout your day are, in my opinion, the best way to start your fitness journey if you haven't already. Even if you have, these are important to add to your day to keep blood flowing and keeping your body happy and healthy. Doing little bits throughout the day in three-to-five--minute bouts four or five times a day is still going to push the needle of fitness and health in the right direction. Just play a song and do something. Walk stairs, sit and stand up from your couch, or just hold some stretches.

MOTIVATION–DISCIPLINE–HABIT: We all start off by needing some motivation. It is usually what gets us started doing something we love. But motivation is not enough to always help us get to where we need to go. We must find a strong "why" and create more discipline, so when motivation isn't there, we have the ability to do what is needed to push us in the right direction. It all starts with one simple step. That can be as basic as putting on your running shoes and going for a walk. If you do this enough time in your life, it will eventually become a habit. It will be just part of who you are and how you function.

GETTING LOVED ONES MOVING: When we genuinely feel good about exercise, we want others to feel the same. It is okay to try to rope in family or friends for a walk or pass a ball around together to try to get them to start. It does come back to how much you know the person. But from my experience, if you lead the way, eventually the people around you will follow. For some people it might take a day, while for others it might take a few years. Some people might be on and off every two to three months, and that's okay because being on sometimes is better than never being on at all. Be the squeaky wheel.

STRESS: Whether it is physical or mental, stress is inevitable. Everyone will all experience it at some point in their lives, whether it is positive or negative. We need to understand what is within our control and focus on that. What human movement does to the brain and body to make us feel better and release stress is not only cool, but for a lot of us, it is a healthy way to manage our daily stressors. Movement will always help other aspects of our lives that makes stress management a little more doable.

SLEEP: This is the best recovery tool we as humans will ever have. Not only will you be a nicer person when you get lots of sleep, you will be more effective in your everyday life. Focus on building a good nighttime routine so you can teach yourself to fall asleep faster and get a good amount of quality sleep so you can crush each day. To those who feel like they need to sacrifice sleep, I suggest you learn to manage your time better instead. You don't want to be that person who stayed up until 3 a.m. studying at the last minute just to fail.

DIET: Food, dieting… these will always be a controversial topic. I will stand by my recommendations of getting an adequate amount of protein, eating a good amount of fruits and vegetables, drinking lots of water, and eating enough to support your lifestyle. Watch out for people who speak in absolutes and those who demonize food. If they are selling you a product and if they are telling you to eat like them to look or feel a certain way, I suggest staying away from that. Always do your own research, but a highly qualified professional is always recommended, unless of course you recognize one of the red flags mentioned above.

FIND WHAT WORKS: The lucky part is that today we have so many options to partake in fitness with our bodies. We can do things like martial arts, gymnastics, and playing soccer or football with our friends. It is important to play and have fun with as many different things as possible. In doing so, you might find the optimum way you enjoy staying fit. This is going to keep you motivated for much longer versus just sticking to one thing in the beginning and potentially realizing you don't like it and stopping altogether.

STRENGTH: If there's one thing every person should do, it's strength training. Strength training at least two to three times a week can provide us with a lifetime of independence, balance, coordination, and the ability to do everyday tasks. Training for strength can come in different forms; it doesn't all have to look the same. As long as you are moving some sort of external load that helps you use the bigger muscles, and you can improve on that over a period of time, you are going to reap the benefits.

BUILDING A HEDGE: As I write this, Eddie had just completed a five-kilometre race for pancreatic cancer. Last year, Eddie walked the race in two hours and two minutes. This year he shaved twenty-three minutes off and completed it in one hour and thirty-nine minutes. The hedge he built before his spinal-cord injury is the reason he can still do what he does. Not everyone has specifics on what they want out of a fitness regime, but one thing we know is that life can throw you a curve ball at any time Aging is inevitable, so build that hedge. That way, we are more resilient when something happens or we get older.

RANGE OF MOTION: Losing range of motion is something that creeps up on us over a long haul. In today's world, we do a lot of things like sit for a prolonged period of time, even though it seemed to be beneficial at first to keep people comfortable. This can hurt us, which is why it is important to pay attention to our bodies and find opposite positions and change positions throughout the day so we can just feel good. A big emphasis is on hips and shoulders as those are our biggest movers, but they are also commonly the regions that get noticeably stiffer over time.

HEALTH MARKERS: Knowing your health markers can have huge benefits as a measuring tool to make sure you are going in the right direction. I used the example of heart rate and blood pressure because those are simple and easy to test on a regular basis. Remember that we, as humans, are resilient. We must respect health markers but not put so much mental energy into them. We must take care of them, but not obsess over them because running, jumping and being independent is where you want to be.

GETTING OFF MEDICATION: We must respect the miracles of medicine and what it does for the human population. Medications are the reason why some people are alive today. However, there are medicines that might be harmful long term and types people use as a quick fix for things like back pain. Improving our health and increasing our general fitness both physically and mentally can help you get off of things like blood pressure medication. If you strengthen your body, you don't have to be as achy during your work shifts. It is all about putting in some work so your body can benefit long term and not rely on a pill.

HOW MUCH SHOULD I TRAIN? There is always so much buzz about more being better and how we need to sacrifice often to achieve results. The truth is that the human body can make incredible adaptions to lots of different stimuli and each of us responds in a different way. Ultimately, as long as you are safe, sleeping well and eating well, you can train quite frequently while managing intensity and safety of whatever it is you are doing. In training for life, what we are looking for is the most sustainable approach to health and fitness over a long haul. That might look very different for each individual, so focus on what you can do.

INJURIES: A lot of people get upset when I tell them it is not a matter of IF you get hurt, but a matter of WHEN. We all experience some sort of injuries in our lives, whether it is from sports, accidents, falls, or in the gym. Training will strengthen your body and increase its ability to become more resilient to injuries and recover better if you do get hurt. We must do what we can to avoid injures, take all the preventative measures, and stay within physiological and psychological tolerances so we can train for tomorrow, not today.

OBSTACLES & CONSISTENCY: It's inevitable that at some point in our lives we will come across obstacles that make fitness drop lower on our priority list. Though, I believe it should never drop, since fitness can help you with so much. Having contingencies can help you overcome some obstacles when it comes to training. Starting a home gym can be a huge step to keeping you consistent and some sort of a community to keep you accountable. Lastly, a solid long-term goal.

GOALS: There are different ways to set goals but having a plan of action is what is most important when it comes to achieving your goals. Using the SMART goals approach is great because it helps lay things out on paper in an organized fashion. Another important point is having distant goals in our heads and understanding that some short-term goals are just that. What matters most is our functionality as a human being when we make our way into old age.

BONUS: CHOOSING A GYM

FOR A LOT OF people, choosing a gym can be intimidating. There are lots of options, depending on where you live, which is why the "finding your style" chapter is so important. You might love one thing and hate the other. When it comes to a conventional gym, you might think of the row of cardio machines, the free-weight section, and the resistance machine section. Nowadays, there are a number of boutique fitness gyms—spin studios, yoga studios, obstacle course-styled playgrounds—and they are all fun. This isn't going to be a description about each one but rather, what should go through your head when deciding what gym is right for you.

Convenience

You're probably going to want to find a place easy to get to so you can make it there on a regular basis, whether on your way to and from work (in my case, the gym is my work). If something is not convenient for you, then the likelihood of excuses for not going starts to ramp up. This is precisely why I recommend people start a home gym EVEN if they are already part of a gym community. It just helps you stay on the path when things get a little rocky.

Community

I am part of a gym where we have group classes and have good relationships between coaches and members. If you can find a place where people care about you, keep you accountable, and it truly feels like a place where you can go to destress, then you've found a good gym. I often say the best coach is the one who cares immensely about the people in front of them, so find yourself a good community. Some of you might not be interested in group-styled training, and that's completely fine. I would still recommend finding a place where the staff clearly cares about the gym they are a part of.

Clean and organized

You should also look for a place where everything is organized and clean. You want to make sure that where you are deciding to sweat and breathe heavily is regularly maintained and cleaned to avoid infections or getting sick. This is also just another way the owners of gyms can show they care about their members. I don't know about you, but I like to tidy my house up a bit before guests come over. I feel like gyms should do the same.

Price

Consider three categories: low, moderate, and high prices.

Low-price gyms: A lot of times, I find that gyms with the lowest usually offer 24/7 service, which is a huge plus for some people. Theoretically, you can go in any time you want. The common issue I find with 24/7 gyms in bigger cities is that they are usually very packed during prime workout hours, and it becomes quite difficult to access some of the equipment. But if you are someone who can workout off prime hours, these gyms can be a great money-saving option. What you really get for a lower price is just the gym. Most cheaper gyms do not have things like a pool, showers, towel services, and all that fun stuff. A lot of these gyms also do not offer personal training, if that is something you are into.

Moderately priced gyms: These are usually those big-box gyms more popular to the public. They have long schedules, but don't always run for 24 hours. Some do, but it is not as common as a lower-priced gym, which might not matter if you plan on working out between 6 a.m. and 11 p.m. A lot of times, these gyms will offer extra amenities, such as showers, blow driers, towel service, and pools or saunas, which are fun once in a while. These gyms usually offer personal training as well, but the option to work out on your own is there. Just like the lower-priced gyms, these still tend to get really busy at peak hours.

Higher-priced gyms: This is typically either a specialized gym or a boutique gym. There are multiple reasons for the high costs here, but I would argue the biggest value offered is because you will be coached through your workout. If you think about spin studios, for example, you don't really have to think: the spin instructor already has a plan for you. These gyms are usually smaller in nature, but there are higher chances of you being able to do a full workout uninterrupted. They don't always offer things like towel service or have pools (some may have it) but it is usually a toss-up because a lot of the higher-priced gyms are typically small businesses. They usually offer personal training and group-styled training, which for these types of gyms means they come with a community and coach (or coaches) that will keep you accountable in the long run.

Home gym: Last, of course, is building your own gym. Start by buying equipment throughout the year—maybe a pair of dumbbells here, you get an ab wheel, and then maybe a spin bike or rower. Before you know it, you've invested that money into your own space and you can do your own thing at home.

My choice: I have seen more consistency and success with people who pay more for their health and fitness. My choice and recommendation if you can afford it, is a gym that offers you a workout, a coach, and a community to guide you through your fitness journey. At the end of the day, treat your health and fitness as an investment. Some people will spend $3 to $5 a day on coffee. That lands anywhere from $90 to $150 a month just on coffee, and let's be real, most of us spend more on other things that do not benefit our health. Remember, building your fitness hedge requires you to start investing now so you can get paid in dividends later, so you should get the best care you can.

You might as well start training for life.

REFERENCES

LONGEVITY

Elmhurst Health. "What your grip strength says about your overall health." Accessed January 25, 2022.
www.eehealth.org/blog/2020/02/
what-your-grip-strength-says-about-your-overall-health.

Harvard Health Publishing. "The Real-World Benefits of Strengthening Your Core." Accessed January 14, 2022.
https://www.health.harvard.edu/healthbeat/
the-real-world-benefits-of-strengthening-your-core.

Health Tide. "The Impact of Leg Strength on Life Expectancy and Brain Health" Accessed January 25, 2022.
https://healthtide.com/impact-leg-strength-life-expectancy-brain-health.

World Health Organization. "GHE: Life Expectancy and Healthy Life Expectancy." Accessed January 14, 2022.
https://www.who.int/data/gho/data/themes/mortality-and-global-health-estimates/
ghe-life-expectancy-and-healthy-life-expectancy.

SLEEP

NHS. "Why lack of sleep is bad for your health." Accessed January 25, 2022.
https://www.nhs.uk/live-well/sleep-and-tiredness/
why-lack-of-sleep-is-bad-for-your-health.

Sleep Foundation. "Caffeine and Sleep. "Accessed January 25, 2022.
https://www.sleepfoundation.org/nutrition/caffeine-and-sleep.

Sleep Foundation. "Sleep Deprivation." Accessed January 25, 2022.
https://www.sleepfoundation.org/sleep-deprivation.

MOVEMENT SNACKS
Centres for Disease Control and Prevention. "How much physical activity do adults
need?" Accessed January 25, 2022
https://www.cdc.gov/physicalactivity/basics/adults/index.htm.

Office of Disease Prevention and Health Promotion. "Top 10 Things to Know About
the Second Edition of the Physical Activity Guidelines for America" Accessed
January 25, 2022.
https://health.gov/our-work/physical-activity/current-guidelines/
top-10-things-know.

GETTING LOVED ONES TO START
TNation. "The "One Lift a Day" Program." Accessed January 25, 2022.
https://www.t-nation.com/workouts/the-one-lift-a-day-program.

STRESS
Centre for Study on Human Stress. "ACUTE VS. CHRONIC STRESS." Accessed January
25, 2022.
https://humanstress.ca/stress/understand-your-stress/acute-vs-chronic-stress.

DIET
CNN, Health. "Twinkie diet helps nutrition professor lose 27 pounds." Accessed
January 25, 2022.
http://www.cnn.com/2010/HEALTH/11/08/twinkie.diet.professor/index.html.

Journal of Translational Medicine. "Intermittent versus continuous energy
restriction on weight loss and cardiometabolic outcomes: a systematic review and
meta-analysis of randomized controlled trials." Accessed January 25, 2022.

https://translational-medicine.biomedcentral.com/articles/10.1186/
s12967-018-1748-4.

National Library of Medicine. "Intermittent energy restriction and weight loss: a
systematic review." Accessed January 25, 2022.
https://pubmed.ncbi.nlm.nih.gov/26603882.

Science Journal. "Daily energy expenditure through the human life course."
Accessed January 25, 2022.
https://www.science.org/doi/10.1126/science.abe5017.

HEALTH MARKERS
Harvard Health Publishing. "What your heart rate is telling you." Accessed January
25, 2022.
https://www.health.harvard.edu/heart-health/what-your-heart-rate-is-telling-you.

WebMD. "5 Heart Rate Myths Debunked." Accessed January 25, 2022.
https://www.webmd.com/heart-disease/features/5-heart-rate-myths-debunked.

GETTING OFF MEDICATION
Lipids in Health and Disease. "Effects of high-intensity circuit training, low-intensity circuit training and endurance training on blood pressure and lipoproteins in
middle-aged overweight men" Accessed January 22, 2022.
https://lipidworld.biomedcentral.com/articles/10.1186/1476-511X-12-131.

ABOUT THE AUTHOR

HERNANI (NANI) OURIQUE, author of *Training for Life,* found his love and passion for fitness and well-being at an early age. Since then, he has spent more than ten years gaining experience in the fitness and health field as a coach and personal trainer, helping people improve their everyday lives. Ourique has expansive knowledge in the fitness and health field, training adaptive clients to elite athletes.

With family as his primary value, Ourique is invested in helping others live long and happy lives, so they can spend as much time as possible with their kids and grandkids for years to come.

Instagram – naniourique
Twitter – naniourique
#trainingforlife

www.ingramcontent.com/pod-product-compliance
Lightning Source LLC
Chambersburg PA
CBHW020324290526
45785CB00007B/2912